# The Therapeutic Pause in Osteopathy and Manual Therapy

## The Somatosensory Integration Time

HANDSPRING
PUBLISHING

EDINBURGH

To my mother

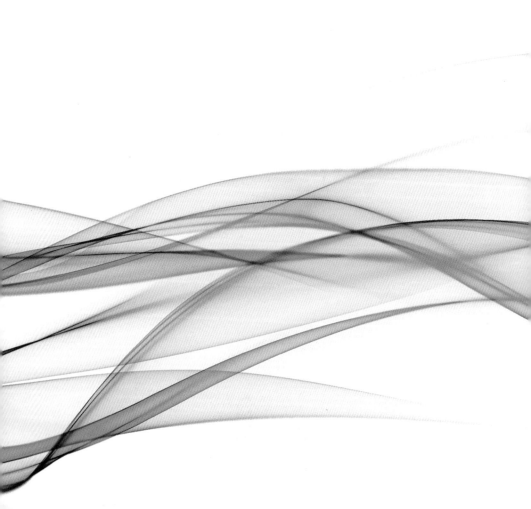

# The Therapeutic Pause in Osteopathy and Manual Therapy

## The Somatosensory Integration Time

### Louise Tremblay

Forewords by
R Paul Lee DO FAAO FCA
and
John Wilks MA RCST BTAA FRSA

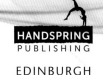

HANDSPRING
PUBLISHING

EDINBURGH

HANDSPRING PUBLISHING LIMITED
The Old Manse, Fountainhall,
Pencaitland, East Lothian
EH34 5EY, United Kingdom
Tel: +44 1875 341 859
Website: www.handspringpublishing.com

First edition published in French, © 2015, Éditions Sully

ISBN 978-1-909141-36-0

**British Library Cataloguing in Publication Data**
A catalogue record for this book is available from the British Library

**Commissioning Editor** Mary Law, Handspring Publishing Limited
**Translation assistance** by Fiona Simpson
**Design direction** by Bruce Hogarth, KinesisCreative
**Cover design** by Bruce Hogarth, KinesisCreative
**Copy editing** by Sally Davies
**Typeset** by DiTech Process Solutions
**Printed** by FINIDR - Czech Republic

The
Publisher's
policy is to use
paper manufactured
from sustainable forests

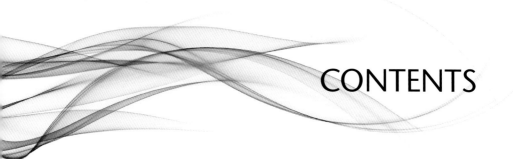

# CONTENTS

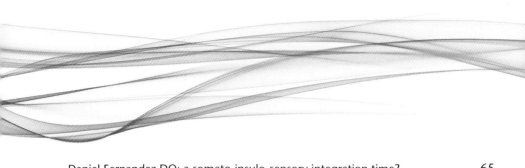

# FOREWORD

"Stillpoint:" a well-known term in osteopathy, signals a deep change and healing during osteopathic treatment. But what is it, really? What varieties does it have? What is its significance? This, and other examples of pauses during treatment, Louise Tremblay discusses in this book in such detail that all who are interested in manual therapy will find it a must read.

In this densely-packed but brief volume, we encounter the function of the insular cortex, how the hypothalamus and thalamus control important homeostatic mechanisms, what the reticular formation does to inhibit an overwhelming amount of external stimuli from becoming conscious, but mostly, we discover in this reading why these and other regions of the neuroendocrine system deserve our attention, as practitioners, to give them some additional time to fully perform their functions. The many neuroendocrine centers deserve ample time, sufficient to complete their complex and interdependent functions. These neuroendocrine functions require more time than it takes to articulate a spinal facet.

Louise Tremblay, in a well-written and easily understood treatise, explains – "gives us pause" – to consider the importance of going slowly, letting the process unfold, allowing it ripen and mature, and giving time for the patient to rest. The level of our success depends upon these considerations.

Often, when I teach students, I mention continuing the treatment until we feel the area of dysfunction become reintegrated into the whole system. In saying this, I believe I am speaking with Louise the language of the body. Waiting for a release is one level of treatment; but treating until the healing effects maximize is another.

Osteopathy is the application of natural principles to effect healing. We feel healing happen under our hands. Observing this process requires one's full attention throughout the unfolding healing events under our hands. Amongst the phenomena that one might observe are pauses, as the body processes and integrates the changes that it is undergoing. These pauses or other changes become landmarks, for the practitioner who is observant, that s/he might follow, patient after patient. We hear the maxim that the patient is the teacher and the osteopath is the student. When we listen to the system in detail, watching for subtle changes, perceiving a density becoming fluid, we tune into the system that heals the body. Healing takes time.

This is not a cookbook explaining a protocol for waiting and watching; rather, it is a thorough analysis of the reasons to do so. There is no recipe for healing. Only the body knows how to do that. We are mere observers of the phenomenon. We must be agile and alert to perceive all that is happening. We must be able to track changes occurring at a distance from our palpating hands. We must be able to think to understand the relationships between the neurology, anatomy and endocrinology. Waiting is an important aspect of this process we call healing.

I learned so much reading Louise's treatise, comprehending the complexities of the neuroendocrine system operating under my therapeutic gaze. I know any manual therapist will find this informative and instructive book an essential read.

R. Paul Lee, DO, FAAO, FCA
Durango, Colorado, USA
August 2015

# FOREWORD

The body appears to naturally demand pauses in the therapeutic process. Our tendency as therapists to want to fix things quickly for a client often overrides this need and so opportunities for the body to respond in its own time are missed. This book is an essential tool for understanding exactly how the body responds to different types of therapeutic touch and why it is so important to allow time for the body to respond.

Pauses can be seen occurring spontaneously in babies and animals when they receive a Bowen treatment. A dog, cat or horse knows instinctively when a pause is necessary, and will often walk away from the therapist to a quiet place for a minute or two, only returning when autonomic and other reactions have settled.

Babies will often display a few moments of stillness as their system responds neurologically to therapeutic touch. During this time many subtle changes are visible as their body responds. The important thing, whether treating animals, babies or adults, seems to be to allow those changes to happen without interruption until their systems have settled and integrated the responses.

There has been considerable debate amongst Bowen therapists as to whether the traditional pauses between moves are really necessary. This book shows conclusively why they are absolutely essential in the therapeutic process.

In craniosacral therapy, watching, waiting and listening are also the cornerstones of treatment. Therapists and clients will often experience periods of 'dynamic stillness', usually within the CV4's or EV4's that Louise Tremblay describes in this book. The power of stillness in allowing the nervous system to settle into these states of deep rest and repair cannot be overstated, and this book explains the process eloquently. For anyone wishing to understand the physiological importance of the therapeutic pause, this book is essential reading.

John Wilks MA RCST BTAA FRSA,
Sherborne, Dorset, UK
September 2015
Author of *Using the Bowen Technique* and
*Choices in Pregnancy and Childbirth*

# PREFACE

Somato-insulo-sensory integration time is a period of time during which the state of apparent immobility of the body allows the sensory stimuli, however minute they may be, to be sent to higher brain centres, and also allows the central nervous system time to react to these stimuli without risk of interference or inhibition from other stimuli. The manual therapist is therefore required to stop during treatment, to make an integration pause, a therapeutic pause, between consecutive stimuli. 'Somato' refers to the fact that some information will reach the somatosensory cortex. 'Insulo' refers to the fact that other information will reach the insular cortex. This depends on which receptors were triggered.

This work was completed initially in May 2009 as a thesis to graduate in osteopathy. For various reasons for the last five years it has remained on the shelf. From time to time, I went back to it and thought we really should do something with it. During the six months I spent writing this thesis, I think I learned more about osteopathy than in the six years of training, and I wanted to go further. It was necessary to bring to the fore this concept of a pause, the effects of which I could see every day in my practice. So I took the thesis off the shelf in March 2014 in order to get back in to it and, as all things are timely, Mr Crepon from Editions Sully wrote to me a few months later to invite me to meet and talk books ... And I found myself back at work, improving, refining and adding comments from two extraordinary osteopaths, Dr Roger Robitaille DO and Dr Francesco Cerritelli DO, who had taken the time to read and mark the 2009 version. Then in 2015 Mary Law from Handspring Publishing kindly agreed to look at this book and we decided to continue the adventure in English.

Perhaps, like good wine, six years in the cellar will have dramatically improved the 2009 version.

It seems that this thesis needed a pause ...

*'Every complex system, whether it's a factory tool or a computer or a human being, has to be congruent. Its parts have to work together; every action has to support every other action if it is to work at a peak level'* (Robbins, 1986, p. 343).

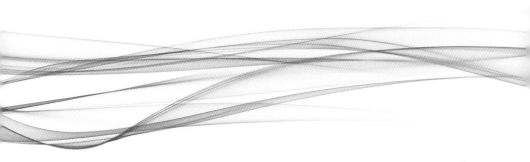

To be true to my life, to all that I am and all that I have learned over years of studying (acupuncture, homeopathy, various manual therapies, and now osteopathy) and dealing with a complex system, I had to find a link which not only unites two inadvertently opposed fields (science and so-called energy treatments),[1] but also draws on the best of both for the benefit of all.

Movement, whether it be vibration, amplitude, oscillation, balancing, flow, a beat, a flux, an impulse, an expansion, a fluctuation, an exchange, etc., is the sign of life. Every human being is animated by these movements, yet no two humans are alike. The same principles of physiology apply to all humans: this is not what differentiates us. We are differentiated by our rhythms and in every rhythm lies a pause.

In recent years we have learned how manual therapies make use of pauses of variable lengths. There is, for example, the 90-second pause used by Dr Jones DO; the 120-second pause in the Bowen technique; and Dr Becker DO and other osteopaths refer to a 'still point.' How can this pause be explained in physiological terms, and how could this pause be integrated into osteopathy?

Deductive and inductive methods are two means of elaborating general knowledge and scientific knowledge in particular. In the deductive method, concepts, definitions, principles, and rules are the starting point, and the goal is to apply these to concrete applications. The inductive method is the inverse: concrete situations which are accessible to the observer are the starting point, and the goal is to identify the applicable concepts, principles or rules from these. Since we are starting with the question *'Would osteopathy benefit from the inclusion of pauses during treatments?'* we must use the inductive method to formulate a principle. This principle could eventually be the basis for research using the deductive method.

Science and medicine view the human being from a particular perspective. The same is true of osteopathy, philosophy and every science that studies humans, whether from up close or from a distance. We must try to distance our perspective in order to recognize better what unites all these visions.

Some criticize science for dividing life up into distinct compartments and therefore forgetting the person as a whole. I am grateful to science for having revealed certain common traits that are shared by all human beings, and for having exposed, analyzed and even compartmentalized them. Once one knows what everyone has in common, one can discern what is particular to the individual. We will therefore refer to current scientific knowledge with a view to understanding the physiology of the pause, and ascertain that it is common among all human beings even if the rhythm is unique to each. Then what do rhythms and integration time mean in osteopathy? Can these two visions be reconciled?

A group of words means nothing if these words are not organized. When they are put in order and given meaning, they become a text, a story. When they are given rhythm, a poem is created.

Rhythm is the poetry of life.

Louise Tremblay

Montreal, 2015

### Note

[1] Osteopathy as an energy treatment as defined by Jean-Pierre Barral, 'The energy theory is that man produces energy, recovers it, and loses it. If these exchanges are harmonious and balanced, the person is in good health. If, on the contrary, the partial or overall energy balance is broken, the person will be ill' (Barral, 2004).

# ACKNOWLEDGEMENTS

Thanks to Dr Roger Robitaille DO for correcting this thesis so well in 2009 ... and in 2014.

Thanks to Dr Francesco Cerritelli DO for revising and correcting all the scientific points and allowing me to discover another aspect of osteopathy linked to scientific research.

Thanks to Fiona Simpson for helping with the translation.

Thanks to Dr Patrick Racano MD for proofreading and corrections.

Thanks to Fiona Rouxel and Lucy Gardner DO for proofreading and corrections.

Thanks to Pierre Saine.

Thanks to my students from whom I learn so much.

Thanks to my children for being there.

All translations are the author's except where otherwise noted.

# INTRODUCTION

*'I began to really progress when I understood that the real question was life and that, osteopathy being a part of life, the best way to understand osteopathy was to understand life'* (Tricot, 2005).

Thus, the osteopath owes it to himself or herself to understand everything that affects humans and their lives. Holistic theory is one of the founding principles of the philosophy of osteopathy. Biology and physiology are only a part of life, albeit an essential part of the knowledge of humans, and therefore of osteopathy. Although pauses have never been particularly emphasized in biology or physiology books, we see that life has many rhythms not limited to movement and which include 'pauses'. Homeostasis is a rhythmic phenomenon as are circadian rhythms, respiratory, cardiac, intestinal, renal and uterine rhythms. Processing of external information, also rhythmic, is transmitted in three steps in order to regulate the internal environment – stimulation, integration and response. Rhythms exist at every level of life.

The period of time between stimulus and integration seems generally to be very short. However, both the time it takes for integration to take place and the period between integration and response vary, sometimes quite substantially.

In music, we say: *'The 'anacrusis' anticipates, the 'crusis' strikes, and the 'metacrusis' receives'* (Sauvanet, 2000). The 'metacrusis' is the pause without which no symphony could exist. Silence allows us to hear.

The objective of this dissertation is to attempt to show that, while osteopathy has developed a complete philosophy with techniques having been recognized countless times for their effectiveness, the field could benefit more from observing other areas of life, including integration time and pauses, or the 'physiological metacrusis'.

One last, important point must be emphasized. For this work, I have referred to the nervous system as it is understood by today's physiologists. It is important that this work be read and accepted by contemporary scientists. Lazorthes tells us that our sensory organs are comparable to slits: They let in only a narrow band of effluvium, light rays, or sound waves. *'The brain is a reductive mechanism that focuses selective atten-*

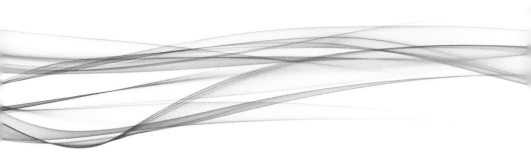

*tion on particular stimuli in order to react in an appropriate manner'* (Lazorthes, 1986).

He also quotes Aldous Huxley, a well-known British author, who compares the brain to a reduction valve that lets only a trickle of reality into its circuit. More importantly, the sensory apparatus does not only include organs that capture stimulations and the pathways that transmit them, but also the specialized areas in the cerebral cortex that perceive them. The specific characteristics and individual capabilities of these vary from one person to another. *'If we could transplant a human eye in another person, that person's eyesight would probably remain unchanged, but he would interpret what was seen differently'* (Lazorthes, 1986).

Here we can identify at least two ideas:

–If our senses are narrow slits which allow only part of reality through, is there another part of reality inaccessible to us?[1] Does this part which is hidden represent a lesser reality or one that is more important? We do not know. It seems to me that we should keep an open and neutral mind when faced with things that appear improbable or impossible to us. Just because we cannot measure a phenomenon doesn't mean that it does not exist.

–This also reminds us that for every osteopath, the interpretation of what he feels in his patient, whether it be a rhythm, fluid or energy expansion, a wave, a tide or no matter what he feels, its interpretation will be slightly (or completely) different from that of another osteopath faced with the same phenomenon.

I will not address the various philosophical interpretations of the phenomena that the osteopath senses. I will try to limit myself to purely 'physiological' considerations and attempt to show that the way in which the nervous system functions validates the importance of pausing during treatments.

Chapter 1, *Speaking the language of the body*, highlights how the nervous system and the endocrine system work, with a physiological reminder of their main functions. Chapter 2, *Homeostasis*, leads us to new concepts of allostasis and limbic touch (or sensual touch). Chapter 3, *The integration time in osteopathy*, is a brief overview, through history, of great osteopaths who already used integration time and how osteopathy approaches, sometimes very closely, somato-insulo-sensory integration time. Chapter 4, *The integration time in other manual therapies*, discusses certain manual therapies where 'pauses' are already emphasized and the reasons behind this. In Chapter 5, *Conceptual analysis*, we will try to define the different types of pause and analyze the merits of using a pause in osteopathy while relating it to the physiology and philosophy of osteopathy.

### Note

[1.] For example, man perceives sounds between 16 Hz and 20,000 Hz. Sounds below 16 Hz are called infrasound and above 20,000 Hz, they are called ultrasound. Some animals, such as the whale, giraffe and elephant, are sensitive to infrasound that our ears cannot hear. Others, such as the dolphin, can hear up to 130,000 Hz. Their reality is very different from ours. Could it be that some people hear infrasound or ultrasound? Could some people be more or less sensitive compared to what is considered 'standard'?

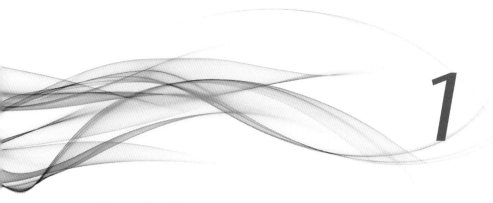

# Speaking the language of the body

Man lives in a state of perpetual interaction with his environment. These interactions not only allow him to move around or react to particular kinds of stimulation, but they are required in order to regulate his internal environment. This requires a constant flow of afferent information, the integration of such information, and feedback response in order to maintain, amongst other things, the optimal state of tension/relaxation of muscle fibers according to the specific requirements and homeostasis in the body; this occurs thanks to the message flow between the various cells of the body. Along with the endocrine system, the nervous system is one of the body's intercellular communication systems.

We communicate. The internal environment and the external environment communicate with the nervous system and the endocrine system, which in turn respond to the internal or the external environment. Where there are feedback messages we call this bidirectional communication.

Osteopathy is a manual therapeutic science founded on an in-depth knowledge of anatomy and physiology among other things. It solicits the body's auto-regulation systems in order to restore harmonious functioning. Working with their hands, osteopaths act on the nervous system, affecting somesthesic afferences, which are the entrances for their influence on the entire body. The term somesthesia means body sensitivity (skin and internal) versus sensory functions (vision, hearing, smell and taste) (Laget, Encyclopédie Universalis, n.d.). For the patient, hearing 'you should relax your arteries because they play an essential part in the normalization of the body,' or seeing a 'released' artery will not solve his problem. The action of the osteopath on the patient is not at the visual or auditory level nor at the sense of taste or smell. Although a patient's intellectual understanding is beneficial to treatment, it is not essential; evidence shows this, and osteopaths working on babies and animals will tell you so. This is *somatosensory* learning. And since the osteopath is seeking self-regulation systems, he must 'speak' the somatosensory language, a language that is perceived, understood and integrated by the central nervous system, which will in turn carry out the desired normalization. Through the somatosensory senses, we can set in motion the process of self-regulation.

We need therefore to understand the basics of how the nervous and endocrine systems work, how they communicate and in what way.

These two systems ensure the coordination of all functions of all body systems.

They are coordinated so that together they make up an integrated super-system called the neuroendocrine system:

–Specific parts of the nervous system stimulate or inhibit the release of hormones that can, in turn, enable or prevent the production of nerve impulses. The nervous system controls muscle contractions and glandular secretions.

–The endocrine system not only helps regulate the actions of smooth muscles, cardiac muscles and certain glands, it also affects just about every other type of tissue.

The nervous, immune and endocrine systems react to stimuli at different rates. In general, nerve impulses have an effect in a few milliseconds. Responses of the endocrine system are often slower than responses of the nervous system; *'although some hormones act within seconds, most take several minutes or more (hours) to illicit a response'* (Tortora and Derrickson, 2009, p. 643). The effects of nervous system activation are generally briefer than those of the endocrine system.

The osteopath must listen to the body's response if he wants to respect the principle of two-way communication. Although we know that the osteopath's action is somatosensory, we do not really know what the response of the nervous system will be: motor, hormonal, or both? It is not in our 'power' to decide how the body will respond. This is also the principle of self-regulation: that is to say that even if the stimulus still comes from the environment (within or external to the body), regulation is by autonomous processes, inherent in the body, *which are not controlled by the environment.*

Although unable to decide on the nature of the nervous system's response, the osteopath can still optimize it if he understands how the treatment center functions, the afferent and efferent pathways, nervous and hormonal.

## Functional components of the nervous system

### *The nervous system*

On the structural level, the nervous system is divided into a peripheral system and a central system The peripheral system is made up of the somatic motor system, which includes the spinal and cranial nerves, and the autonomic nervous system (ANS), which is subdivided into the sympathetic system (which incites prompt reactions in the body), the parasympathetic system (which tends to protect and relax the body) and an enteric nervous system sometimes called 'the second brain' due to its independence from the central nervous system (CNS). Gershon (1998) provides a useful explanation of the enteric nervous system:

> The enteric nervous system, uniquely, can escape from the functional hierarchy of the CNS. Technically, the enteric nervous system is a component of the peripheral nervous system, but it is so only by definition. The enteric nervous system does not necessarily follow commands it receives from the brain or spinal cord; nor does it inevitably send the information it receives back to them. The enteric system is not a slave of the brain but a contrarian, independent spirit in the nervous organization of the body. It is a rebel, the only element of the peripheral nervous system that can elect not to do the bidding of the brain or spinal cord.

The ANS is not completely peripheral because it is managed by centers located in the CNS, in particular the hypothalamus, which is the main regulator of the autonomic preganglionic neurons.

Together, the somatic motor system and the ANS constitute the total neural output of the CNS. The somatic motor system has one single function: it innervates and commands skeletal muscle fibers. The ANS has the complex task of commanding every other innervated tissue and organ in the body (Bear, Connors and Paradiso, 2007, p. 492).

From a schematic point of view, we could say that the central system is made up of the following (Fig. 1.1):

1. the spinal cord;

2. the brainstem, which is composed of the medulla oblongata, the pons, the cerebellum, and the mesencephalon;

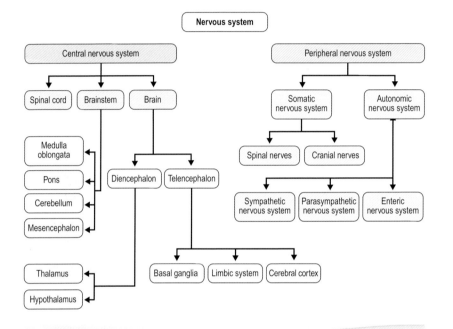

**FIGURE 1.1**

Organization of the nervous system

3. the brain, which is composed of the diencephalon and the telencephalon, including:

– the thalamus, the hypothalamus;

– the basal ganglia, the limbic system and the cerebral cortex.

The nervous system carries out three functions (Fig. 1.2):

–The sensory system is responsible for conveying the information coming from the environment to the nerve centers, with help from the afferent neurons.

–The motor system is involved, through efferent neurons, in the transmission, toward effectors, of commands programed in the nerve centers.

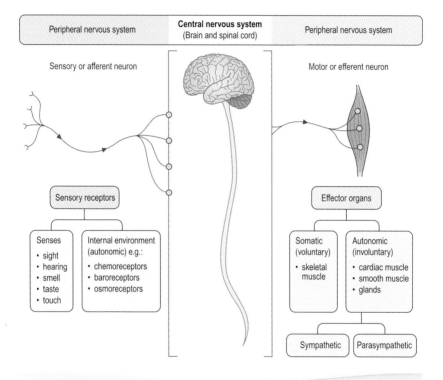

**FIGURE 1.2**

Functional components of the nervous system. Reproduced with permission from Waugh and Grant, Anatomy and physiology in health and illness. p. 138. Elsevier 2010.

—As for treatment centers, they are made up of circuits composed mainly of interneurons, and their function is to process information and program reactions.

### The nerve impulse

The nerve impulse that travels along the neurons is the basis of the information transmitted to the nerve centers for processing. These nerve impulses, which are passing through billions of nerve fibers, are not different from one another, regardless of the type of information they are transmitting. Why do we hear sounds through the ears and see objects or colors through the eyes, not the other way around? Simply because the difference between the messages is not created by the message itself, but by its destination. If a muscle is the destination, the muscle will contract or relax. If a gland is the destination, it will accelerate, slow down or stop secreting. If the destination is one part of the brain an image will appear, and if it is another part of the brain the message will be decoded as a sound. '*Ultimately*, says Godefroid, *we would only have to rewire the nerves, connecting the optic nerve to the part of the brain that analyzes sound in order for the visual information captured by the eyes to be heard*' (Godefroid, 2008, p. 175).

The overall organization of the three main types of exit from the central nervous system is illustrated in Figure 1.3.

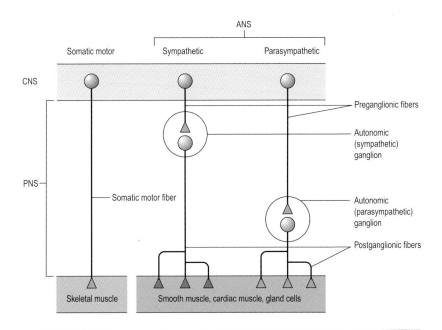

**FIGURE 1.3**

The organization of the three neural outputs of the CNS. Reproduced with permission from Bear, Connors and Paradiso, 2007, p. 492

1.  The sole output of the somatic motor system is by the lower motor neurons in the ventral horn of the spinal cord and the brainstem, which Sherrington[1] called the final common pathway for the generation of behavior (Bear, Connors and Paradiso, 2007, p. 492).

2.  But some behavior, such as salivating, sweating, and genital stimulation, depends instead on the ANS. These visceral motor responses are dependent on the sympathetic system and the parasympathetic divisions of the ANS, whose lower motor neurons (i.e., postganglionic neurons) lie outside the CNS in autonomic ganglia (Bear, Connors and Paradiso, 2007, p. 492).

The 'second brain,' as the enteric division of the ANS is sometimes called, is a unique neural system embedded in an unlikely place: the lining of the oesophagus, stomach, intestines, pancreas, and gallbladder. The enteric system is not small; it contains about the same number of neurons as the entire spinal cord! (See Bear, Connors and Paradiso, 2007, p. 495.) The enteric nervous system receives input from the parasympathetic and sympathetic parts of the nervous system, and the gastrointestinal tract also receives a plentiful supply of afferent nerve fibers, through the vagus nerves and spinal afferent pathways. Thus, there is a rich interaction, in both directions, between the enteric nervous system, the sympathetic prevertebral ganglia and the CNS (Furness, 2007).

### The law of all or nothing

Neither the stimulus received from the environment nor its energy is carried along the dendrites and the axons. A stimulus only transforms the potential for rest in the extremities of the dendrites of a receptor into a potential for action that then travels through the axon, little by little, through a series of successive depolarizations called pulse trains. Since each fiber has its own electrical potential, the propagated impulse remains unchanged, whatever the intensity or the characteristics of the stimulus. This means that the impulse will only be released at dendrite level if the activation, provoked by the stimulation of a receptor or the arrival of an impulse originating from another neuron, is great enough to break through its threshold. Anything less and nothing will happen: This is the law of all or nothing (Godefroid, 2008, p. 175).

*1*

The osteopath is called upon to act on the body through the somatosensory afferent pathways, known formerly as afferent pathways of the sense of touch. These use the same mode of transmission of nerve impulses as all other pathways coming from the sense of sight, hearing, taste or smell.

Sensitivity to various stimuli varies between sensory receptors (a hearing receptor will not be stimulated by light, for example), but each of these receptors has the ability to transform a particular stimulus into a nerve impulse by a transduction mechanism inherent in each type of receptor (see 'Afferents: sensitive sensory receptors', p. 18).

Somatosensory receptors are not all susceptible to the same types of stimulation; however, all stimuli must cross the targeted receptor threshold for it to react.

The manual therapist must be aware of these differences in order to stimulate what he wants to stimulate in the patient and how to go about it.

Scientific research is quite precise regarding afferents (although research is ongoing at this level), how receptors work, and how impulses reach the CNS by ascending pathways. Less understood, however, is the scope of the CNS response to stimulation. Indeed, *all efferent nerve impulses fall on skeletal muscles, smooth muscles or glands through the ANS, or more likely all of them at the same time. We are not able to control or limit the scope of the response from the CNS.*

Thus, the therapist offers ... and the body has the means.

## Different neural systems generate different responses

Most neural systems are organized anatomically to the extent that we can see a 'point-to-point' relationship from one neuron to another (as shown in Fig. 1.4A). The proper functioning of these systems requires restricted synaptic activation of target cells and signals of brief duration. In contrast, three other components of the nervous system act over great distances and for long periods of time (Fig.1.4B). Neurons of the secretory hypothalamus affect their many targets by releasing hormones directly into the bloodstream (Fig. 1.4C). Networks of interconnected

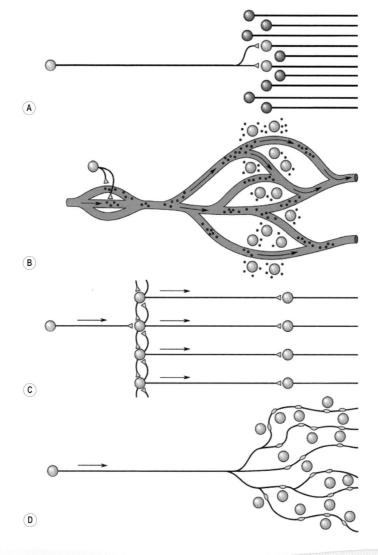

**FIGURE 1.4**

Patterns of communication in the nervous system. Reproduced with permission from Bear, Connors and Paradiso, 2007, p. 483

neurons of the ANS can work together to activate tissues all over the body (Fig. 1.4D). Diffuse modulatory systems extend their reach with widely divergent axonal projections. The diffuse systems are believed to regulate, among other things, the level of arousal and mood.

### Prolongation of the postdischarge signal

*An example of the point-to-point relationship of neuronal systems: the reverberating circuit, a feedback loop that takes its time ...*

The CNS contains billions of neurons organized into complicated networks called neural circuits – functional groups of neurons that process specific types of information. In a simple series circuit, a presynaptic neuron stimulates a single postsynaptic neuron. The second neuron then stimulates another, and so on. However, most neural circuits are more complex (Tortora and Derrickson, 2009, p. 451).

A signal entering one or a group of neurons causes a prolonged discharge (called postdischarge) which lasts a few milliseconds to several minutes after the end of the afferent signal (Fig. 1.5). This postdischarge mechanism, which is called a reverberating (or oscillatory) circuit, prolongs the signal. These reverberating or oscillatory circuits are some of the most important circuits of the nervous system. They are maintained by positive feedback within the neuronal network. The signal emitted at the exit of the neural circuit re-excites the signal at the entrance to the same circuit.

This type of circuit is found in the larger networks (such as the reticular formation (Vibert, 2007, p.9)) where many connections ensure that, after a variable delay, the signal returns to its emitter.

Once stimulated, the circuit fires repeatedly in a feedback loop for a moment. *'The input stimulus may last only one millisecond or so, and yet the output can last for many milliseconds or even many minutes'* (Hall and Guyton, 2011, p. 567). Tortora and Derrickson state: 'The output signal may last from a few seconds to many hours, depending on the number of synapses and the arrangement of neurons in the circuit. Inhibitory neurons may turn off a reverberating circuit after a period of time' (2009, p. 452).

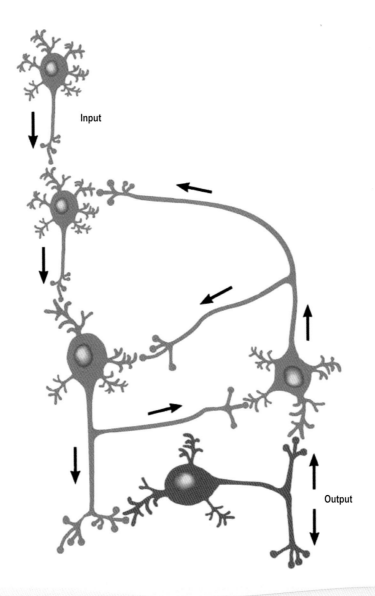

Input

Output

**FIGURE 1.5**
Reverberating circuit. Reproduced with permission from Tortora and Grabowski, 2001, p. 426

The duration of the total signal before cessation can be controlled by signals from other parts of the brain that inhibit or facilitate the circuit.

The autonomic nervous system uses this type of information transmission to control functions such as vascular and intestinal tone, the constriction of the iris and heart rate. 'Also, among the body responses thought to be the result of output signals from reverberating circuits, are breathing, coordinated muscular activities, waking up, and short-term memory' (Tortora and Derrickson, 2009, p. 452).

*... and, after a certain point, exhausts itself to the point of ineffectiveness.*

'Almost every part of the brain is directly or indirectly interconnected with the other parts, which poses a serious problem. If the first part excites the second, and the second the third and so on until finally the signal once again excites the first part, it is clear that an excitatory signal in any part of the brain would set off a continuous cycle of re-excitation in all parts. If this should occur, the brain would be inundated by a mass of uncontrolled reverberating signals that would be transmitting no information but, nevertheless, would be consuming the circuits of the brain, making it impossible for any other information signals to be transmitted. One of the mechanisms that prevent this phenomenon from occurring is synaptic fatigue: a progressive weakening of the synaptic transmission that continues as long as the excitation period continues. [The other mechanism is an inhibitor signal originating from different parts of the brain.] Consider, as an example, the study of an animal's flexion reflex as provoked by a painful stimulus in the pad of the paw. The strength of the contraction diminishes progressively with each take. It is thought that the fatiguing of synapses in the flexion reflex circuit causes this diminishment. The shorter the interval between successive flexion reflexes is, the lower the intensity of the reflex response' (Hall and Guyton, 2011 p. 569).

This phenomenon occurs in many cerebral pathways. Those that are often over-used become fatigued and their potential is thus diminished; whereas those that are under-used relax, and their sensitivity increases. *'Thus, fatigue and recovery from fatigue constitute an important short-term means of moderating the sensitivity of the different nervous system circuits. These help to keep the circuits operating in a range of sensitivity that allows effective function'* (Hall and Guyton, 2011 p. 569).

It is important to allow neural circuits a recovery time. Perhaps we find here one of the reasons that could tend to favor somato-insulo-sensory integration time?

The concept of synaptic plasticity has been widely studied by neuroscience in recent decades. Joseph LeDoux (2002) says, *'Most brain systems are plastic, modifiable by experience, which means that synapses involved will change through experience.'*

In Appendix I we find further explanation regarding the phenomenon of habituation and how it is reversible through the plasticity of synapses.

### The hormonal pathway

Endocrine control is mostly ensured by the secretions produced by the pituitary gland (the main endocrine gland that is attached to the nerve centers, principally to the hypothalamus situated at the base of the brain). Although the hypothalamus is classified as a part of the brain and not as an endocrine gland, it controls the pituitary gland and has an indirect effect on many other glands.

The pituitary gland is made up of an anterior and a posterior lobe, each of which is controlled in a very different manner by the hypothalamus, which is connected to them by the pituitary stalk:

> The largest of the hypothalamic neurosecretory cells, magnocellular neurosecretory cells, extend axons around the optic chiasm, down the stalk of the pituitary, and into the posterior lobe of the pituitary gland (Fig. 1.6). The magnocellular neurosecretory cells release two neurohormones into the bloodstream: oxytocin, which stimulates contractions in the uterus during labor and orgasm and the release of milk during breastfeeding; and vasopressin, or anti-diuretic hormone (ADH) which regulates blood volume and salt concentration.

> The anterior lobe is under the control of neurons in the periventricular area called parvocellular neurosecretory cells. These hypothalamic neurons do not extend axons all the way into the anterior lobe; instead, they communicate with their targets via the bloodstream (Fig. 1.7).

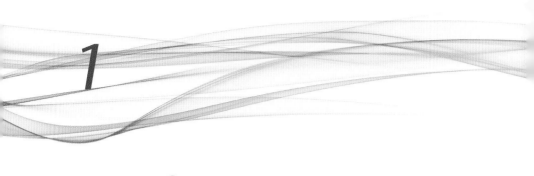

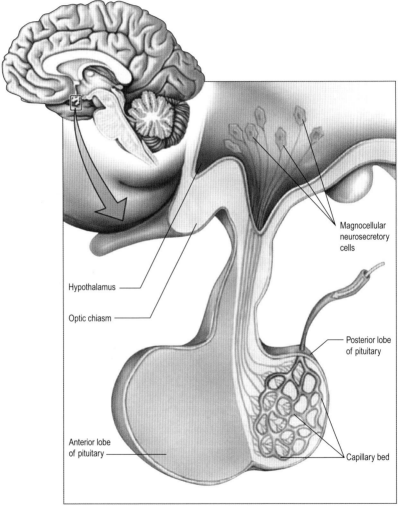

**FIGURE 1.6**

Magnocellular neurosecretory cells of the hypothalamus. Reproduced with permission from Bear, Connors and Paradiso, 2007, p. 486

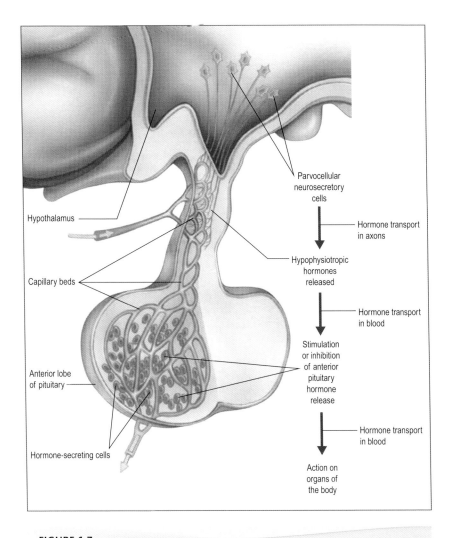

**FIGURE 1.7**

Parvocellular neurosecretory cells of the hypothalamus. Reproduced with permission from Bear, Connors and Paradiso, 2007, p. 489

These neurons secrete what are called hypophysiotropic hormones (also called releasing hormones or RH hormones) into the hypothalamopituitary portal circulation. Hypophysiotropic hormones, secreted by hypothalamic neurons into the portal circulation, travel downstream until they bind to specific receptors on the surface of pituitary cells. Activation of these receptors causes the pituitary cells to either secrete or stop secreting hormones into the general circulation. (Bear, Connors and Paradiso, 2007, p. 485)

'The endocrine system is a control system whose function is similar to that of the nervous system. Both help balance the internal environment, whilst influencing growth, development, reproduction and other body functions. Whereas the nervous system uses neurotransmitters to transmit nerve impulses, the endocrine system transmits its messages through hormones.

'The other endocrine glands are located in various parts of the body. They can be divided into three groups: a group whose hormones regulate nutritional functions and metabolic processes, the basis of homeostasis; a second group to monitor reproductive functions; and a third group whose secretions intervene in emergency situations' (Godefroid, 2008, p. 182).

Following stimulation, the hypothalamus sends a message to either the posterior pituitary gland or the anterior pituitary gland in order to regulate the hormonal balance of the body (see 'Information processing', p. 27).

*'Responses of the endocrine system often are slower than responses of the nervous system; although some hormones act within seconds, most take several minutes or more to cause to a response. The effects of the nervous system activation are generally briefer then those of the endocrine system'* (Tortora and Derrickson, 2009, p. 643).

### The interconnected neural networks in the ANS

'Besides controlling the ingredients of the hormonal soup that flows in our veins, the periventricular zone of the hypothalamus also controls the autonomic nervous system (ANS). The ANS is an extensive network of interconnected neurons that are widely distributed inside the body cavity. From the Greek *autonomia*, autonomic roughly means 'independence'; autonomic functions are usually carried out automatically, without conscious, voluntary control. They are also highly coordinated functions.

'Some behavior, such as salivating, sweating, and genital stimulation, depends instead on the ANS. These visceral motor responses depend on the sympathetic and parasympathetic divisions of the ANS, whose lower motor neurons (i.e., postganglionic neurons) lie outside the CNS in autonomic ganglia.

'The physiological influences of the sympathetic and parasympathetic divisions generally oppose each other. The sympathetic division tends to be most active during a crisis, real or perceived (fight, flight or fright). The parasympathetic division facilitates various processes, such as digestion, growth, immune responses, and energy storage. In most cases, the activity levels of the two ANS divisions are reciprocal; when one is high, the other tends to be low, and vice versa. The sympathetic division frenetically mobilizes the body for a short-term emergency at the expense of processes that keep it healthy over the long term. The parasympathetic division works calmly for long-term well-being. Both cannot be stimulated strongly at the same time; their general goals are incompatible. Fortunately, neural circuits in the CNS inhibit activity in one division when the other is active' (Bear, Connors and Paradiso, 2007, p. 490).

### The diffuse modulatory systems of the brain

'The brain has several collections of neurons, each using a particular neurotransmitter and making widely dispersed, diffuse, almost meandering connections. Rather than carrying detailed sensory information, these cells often perform regulatory functions, modulating vast assemblies of postsynaptic neurons (such as the cerebral cortex, the thalamus, and the spinal cord) so that they become more or less excitable, more or less synchronously active, and so on. Collectively, they are a bit like the volume, treble, and bass controls on a radio, which do not change the lyrics or melody of a song but dramatically regulate the impact of both. In addition, different systems appear to be essential for aspects of motor control, memory, mood, motivation, and metabolic state' (Bear, Connors and Paradiso, 2007, p. 498).

*1*

### Summary

Let us say that once activated the brain will respond, regardless of the stimulation. It will respond differently, of course, depending on the type of stimulation and the impact produced by it. But it will take one path, or another, or more than one path in order to adapt constantly to stimuli. It is the function of the CNS: to ensure that at any time, in any place, the body can adapt and evolve ... or adapt and survive.

*Whilst knowing that there will be a CNS response, the manual therapist cannot know whether it will be hormonal, circuit reverberating or another response. But he knows that no matter what the type of response, it can be inhibited ... perhaps by other stimuli?*

## Afferents: sensitive sensory receptors

As stated earlier, the osteopath's entire being, the hands in particular, is used to help the patient's entire being. This is done for the most part through the somesthesic pathway.

To duplicate anatomy with his hands is a part of the osteopath's work; understanding and sensing how the impact of our actions unfolds is also essential. We work with sensitive tools. Let us try to understand what is common to all those receptors.

### Transduction

A physical stimulus is 'translated' into a sensory signal in the sensory organs. The process whereby a stimulus connected with the environment causes a variation of potential in a sensory receptor cell is called transduction. The numerous transduction mechanisms of the nervous system make it sensitive to, among other things, chemical substances, pressure, sound, and light. The nature of the transduction mechanism determines the specific sensitivity of the sensory system. A sensory receptor, whether it is in the retina, the cochlea, or taste buds, is formed from a group of highly specialized nerve cells. Through transduction, these cells transform part of the energy present in the environment in the form of photons, moving air molecules, scent molecules or sapid molecules, etc., into neuronal impulses which carry information about that stimulation to the brain through the afferent fibers of the cranial and spinal nerves. So they are able to translate a physical signal into a language understandable to the CNS.

## Sensory modalities

In Chapter 2, we will study a new classification of sensory modalities developed by Dr Craig (2015): interoception and exteroception. At this stage, we will use the usual classification as outlined below.

'In general, classification of sensory modalities is as follows: vision, hearing, touch[2] taste and smell. There are many others, such as sensitivity to heat and cold, pain, and those for the most part unconscious sensory modalities that inform the central nervous system of the composition or state of the internal environment.' As, for example, the chemoreceptors which detect oxygen level in the arterial blood or the electromagnetic receptors which detect light on the retina of the eye (Hall and Guyton, 2011, p. 559).

'The term 'general somatosensory sensitivity' refers to the conscious sensations aroused by stimulation of body tissue; sensations that are neither visual nor auditory; neither taste nor smell. They are caused by the excitation of receptor nerve endings of various types, located in the surface of the skin and some deeper tissue: the visceral connections, capsules and ligaments of the joints. These receptors are sensitive to a number of specific stimulants: mechanical, thermal, painful. Within somesthesia we can therefore distinguish tactile, thermal and painful sensitivity, and also kinaesthetic awareness, which comes from joints and provides information about the position and movements of various body segments in space' (Laget, Encyclopédie Universalis, n.d.).

All manual therapies have an effect on somesthesia receptors. According to the techniques used, different receptors are more or less stimulated but good stimulation will affect the desired receptor, and it is up to the therapist to choose the stimulation which is best for the patient.

## Contrast detectors

Sensory systems are contrast detectors. Contrast represents the ratio of intensity of two adjacent stimulations. ***Whatever the sensory modality,*** *two stimulations can only be perceived if there is a contrast between them* (Rose, 2004). The differential threshold is the minimal difference in amplitude required in order to differentiate two stimuli. The reinforcement of the contrast between two closely placed stimulations is an important attribute of all sensory systems.

A uniformly grey stripe (Fig. 1.8 in the middle) appears darker on the left and lighter on the right because it is framed by two stripes of graduated washes that are lighter on the left and darker on the right.

At the somesthesic level, we can consider the example of clothing we are wearing that we no longer 'feel' after a few seconds of our having put it on, the contrasts being too weak to 'draw the attention' of the CNS. It is the same for the osteopath's hands. When he places his hands, and is in listening mode, he induces nothing in the tissue but seeks to feel[3]. While the osteopath places his hands, and is in listening mode, inducing nothing in the tissue but only seeking to feel, the patient's somatosensory receptors are no longer stimulated. The period of time that the osteopath keeps his hands in place and waits, for example, for the sign of a 'great tide', as will be discussed further when we consider Becker, is a somato-insulo-sensory therapeutic pause. No contrast (or very little) is perceived by the patient's somatosensory receptors, no action potential is transmitted to the brain via the nerve fibers. The

**FIGURE 1.8**
Apparent contrast between two adjacent stimulations

normalization which results in changes perceivable to the osteopath, depending on whether it is mechanical, nervous or hormonal, may take a few milliseconds, seconds, or a few minutes to occur, or even a few hours, days, or weeks, and the osteopath cannot keep his hands in place all this time. However, we can say that as long as the osteopath is listening, his somesthesic senses are at the highest level of vigilance: the slightest contrast in his hands will inform him of the patient's state.

Black is especially visible on a white background, not so much on a dark blue background. Sounds are clear if they are not lost amongst other noise. The therapeutic pause could well be the contrast needed for somato-insulo-sensory inputs.

### The physiological and perceptive thresholds

The body collects information on two levels: at the lower level, every event that has the necessary characteristics and enough energy to excite a receptor brings about the production of a coded message that will be transmitted to the brain. The minimum limit of sensitivity of each sensory organ below which no excitation can take place is called the physiological threshold. At the superior level, the information received with each perception must cross another threshold, the perceptive threshold of conscious recognition which is controlled by the reticular formation (see 'Information processing', p. 27).

*In other words, even if the physiological threshold of excitation is reached, as long as the perceptive threshold is not reached, the stimulation will not be perceived.*

### The relation between stimulus intensity and the receptor potential

In general, the frequency of repetitive action potentials transmitted from sensory receptors increases approximately in proportion to the increase in receptor potential. Even if a weak sensory stimulation can provoke at least some signal, very intense stimulation of the receptors provokes a proportionally decreasing increase in numbers of action potentials. This is an exceedingly important principle that is applicable to almost all sensory receptors. It allows the receptor to be sensitive to very weak sensory experiences and yet not reach a maximum firing rate until the sensory experience is extreme (Hall and Guyton, 2011, p. 561).

Thus, for instance, at weak levels the Pacinian corpuscles are capable of precisely measuring extremely minimal changes in the intensity of a stimulus. However, with greater intensities, the change must be much greater in order to provoke an identical change in the receptor potential.

*Therefore, the greater the stimulus, the greater its variation must be in order for the brain to detect it.*

### Receptor adaptation

At any given time, the sensory receptors are flooded with stimuli to the point that the brain, which processes them, would be at risk of being plunged into a state of informational overload if it were not for the regulatory mechanisms that maintain the quantity of stimuli at a more or less constant level that is acceptable for the body (Godefroid, 2008, p. 286).

The most important of these mechanisms is sensory adaptation, which consists of the sensory system's tendency to react less and less to continuous or repeated exposure to a stimulus (Godefroid, 2008, p. 290).

Thus, another characteristic of all sensory receptors is that they adapt either partially or completely to any constant stimulus after a period of time. That is, when a continuous sensory stimulus is applied, the receptors respond initially at a high response rate and then at a progressively slower rate until finally the rate of action potentials decreases to very few or often to none at all (Hall and Guyton, 2011, p. 562).

The degree to which adaptation occurs varies from one sense to another. Some touch receptors (Meissner's and Pacinian corpuscles) will adapt rapidly while spindle cells and pain receptors will adapt slowly. There appears to be an advantage in this. Light touch could be distracting if it were persistent; and, conversely, slow adaptation of spindle cells (the type II fibers) is needed to maintain posture (Barrett et al., 2010, p. 153). Type Ia fibers of the muscle spindle are those which are sensitive to a sudden and rapid stretching of the muscle spindle and are responsible for the dynamic stretch reflex. This reflex stops for a split second after stretching the muscle. Type II fibers of the muscle spindle are responsible for the static stretch reflex. This reflex maintains the degree of contraction of the muscle for at least several seconds or minutes. The receptor continues to send its signals as the muscle spindle is stretched.

*'Sensory adaptation is a useful adaptive mechanism for the body which becomes better able to detect and focus on any change or any development occurring in its environment'* (Godefroid, 2008, p. 290).

### Summary

Conditions exist so that information, somatosensory or other, is led to processing centers, that is to say the CNS.

Firstly, the right stimulation to the right receptor is required so that it can transform the information into nerve impulses through its transduction capacity.

Next, if we want to influence a deep-touch receptor, we do not remain too superficial or light. This means that we must reach the physiological threshold of the receptor to switch it on. Once this threshold is reached, we avoid intensifying the stimulation so that subsequent stimulations are just as perceivable without increasing (or greatly increasing) the intensity of that stimulation.

Next, it seems preferable to 'create' a contrast so that the proposed information has more opportunity to be perceived by the CNS. This contrast could be an important element in preventing the receptors from adapting.

Finally, we must reach the perceptual threshold, that is to say, the filter of the reticular formation, so that information goes to the data center.

### Afferents: the somesthesic system

When the proposed information has responded well to the activation criteria and is moving toward the processing centers, it must take one of two pathways: the dorsal column pathway or the anterolateral pathway of the spinal cord (Fig. 1.9).

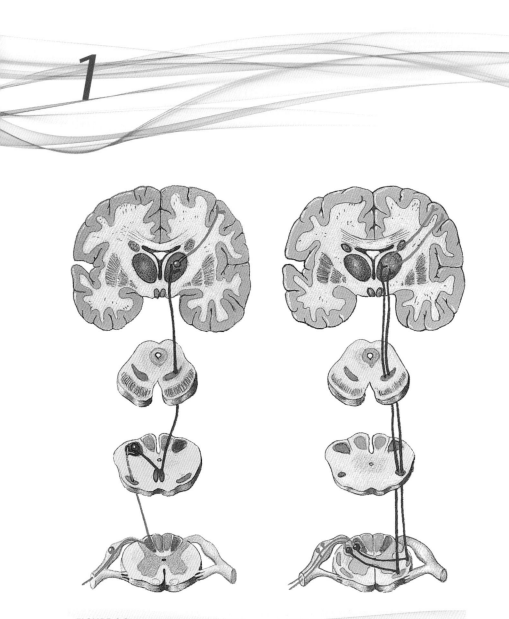

**FIGURE 1.9**

The dorsal column–medial lemniscus pathway and the spinothalamic tract. Reproduced with permission from Tortora and Grabowski, 2001, p. 521

The somesthesis system is sensitive to many kinds of stimuli: the pressure of objects against the skin, the position of joints and muscles, distension of the bladder, and the temperature of the limbs and of the brain itself. Its receptors are distributed throughout the body rather than being concentrated at small, specialized locations. Because it responds to many different kinds of stimuli, we can think of it as a group of at least four senses rather than a single one: the senses of touch, temperature, pain, and body position. In fact, those four can in turn be subdivided into many more. The somatic sensory system is really a catch-all name, a collective category for all the sensations that are not seeing, hearing, tasting, smelling, and the vestibular sense of balance (Bear, Connors and Paradiso, 2007, p. 388).

The somatosensory system is the only sensory system which is not located only at head-level; it spreads over the entire body, completely covering the external and internal surfaces.

As we will see in the next chapter, the somatosensory system can be divided into exteroceptive somatosensory afferents using the mechanoreceptors and interoceptive somatosensory afferents which use primary afferent A∂ and C-type fibers.

### The two sensory transmission paths taken by somatic signals to the central nervous system

Almost all sensory information from the somatic segments of the body enters the spinal cord through the dorsal roots of the spinal nerves. However, from entry points into the cord and then to the brain, the sensory signals are carried through one of two alternative sensory pathways: 1) the dorsal column–medial lemniscal system or 2) the spinothalamic tract–extralemniscal system (Hall and Guyton, 2011, p. 573). These two systems come back together partially at the level of the thalamus (Fig. 1.9) and then to the cerebral cortex only if the information carried by the sensory pathways passes through the filter of the reticular formation, which only allows stimuli that are particularly useful or intense to arrive at the level of consciousness (see 'The reticular formation', p. 27).

The dorsal column or lemniscal system transmits information that must be transmitted rapidly with temporal and spatial fidelity. Information that does not require rapid transmission or great spatial fidelity is transmitted mainly by the extralemniscal system or spinothalamic tract.

Thus, the first is restricted to the finest mechanical sensations (information which requires great temporal and spatial fidelity):

–touch sensations requiring a high degree of localization of the stimulus;

–touch sensations requiring transmission of fine gradations of intensity;

–phasic sensations such as vibratory sensations;

–sensations that signal movement against the skin;

–position sensations from the joints;

–pressure sensations related to fine degrees of judgement of pressure intensity.

The second is limited to interoceptive sensations (see 'The sensual touch', Chapter 2, p. 40):

–pain;

–thermal sensations, including both warm and cold sensations;

–crude touch and pressure sensation only capable of crude localization on the surface of the body;

–tickle and itch sensations;

–sexual sensations;

–sensual (or limbic) touch.

All sensory signals, not only those that are somesthesic in origin, must clear the filter of the reticular formation before they can reach the thalamus and, eventually, the cerebral cortex (see 'The reticular formation', p. 27).

## Information processing

Thus, there is an entry point, an exit point and between these an information processing and reaction-programming center. It is during this stage of information processing and reaction programming that the nature of the response will be determined.

## The activating systems of the brain

The brain would be unusable without the continuous transmissions of nerve signals it receives from the brainstem. Severe compression of the brainstem, as sometimes results from a pineal tumor, often causes the person to go into an unremitting coma. Nerve signals in the brainstem activate the cerebral part of the brain in two ways: by directly stimulating a background level of neuronal activity in wide areas of the brain (the reticular formation and the thalamus) or by activating neurohormonal systems that release specific facilitatory or inhibitory hormone-like neurotransmitter substances into selected areas of the brain (Hall and Guyton, 2011, p. 711).

### The reticular formation

The reticular formation is the major center which controls the overall level of brain activity (alertness). It is important to understand its role and functions. By studying and better understanding this part of the brain, one approaches the true language of the body.

A very good description of the reticular formation can be found on the website 'les neurobranchés' (Rose, 2004):

> The reticular formation is a long column of nerve tissue which extends from the cervical cord to the diencephalon. It is in the center of the brainstem. It consists of a very dense network of fibers in mesh in which there are a large number of cells, some of which are grouped into blocks and form nuclei. It forms a nonspecific, very complex multi-synaptic network, located at the crossroads of the three major systems: sensory, motor and autonomic.

> It is the headquarters of a surprising convergence of afferent impulses from receptors of all kinds, located in all parts of the body. The same reticular cell can be activated by auditory, visual and tactile stimuli from several cutaneous areas. In the reticular system, the specificity of sensory modalities of related messages disappears.

*The role of reticular cells is to integrate the intensity of nerve signals which converge there, whatever the origin of these messages.*

*If the reticular activating system makes the individual more attentive to a given stimulus, it simultaneously reduces the access to the cortex of sensory messages from other origins through inhibition of the corresponding sensory pathways.*

*It causes a parallel synaptic facilitation of short duration in the optic tract, a facilitation that accompanies, under physiological conditions, the attention reaction which is triggered by unexpected stimuli.*

*It finally prepares the subject to respond to stimulation, by facilitating the control of effector muscles. It also works at motor level, playing a large role in the control of posture and balance.*

Let's add the role of the reticular formation in large vegetative regulation. It certainly coordinates the activity of the cranial nerve nuclei and thus is involved in highly complex functions such as breathing, coughing, sneezing, control of the cardiovascular system, swallowing and vomiting, and phonation.

'It is the activity of the reticular formation which determines the level of general activity of the nervous system and the body. According to this level of activity, information will be treated differently.

We saw earlier that the physiological threshold was this limit of sensitivity of each sense organ without which neuronal excitation cannot take place. And also at a higher level, in order to be perceived, the information has to cross another threshold, called the perceptual threshold, which is that of conscious recognition and which is controlled by the reticular formation. Thus, the information will reach the cortex and consciousness if it is deemed appropriate by the centers of the reticular formation.

*The ascending reticular activating system seems to serve as a filter for this influx of sensory information. It weakens repetitive, familiar or weak signals but allows unexpected, important or intense signals to reach the consciousness.*

*'The ascending reticular activating system and the cerebral cortex no doubt neglect 99% of the sensory stimuli registered by our receptors'* (Marieb, 1993, p. 401).

The neurons of the reticular formation reconnect with the cells of the hypothalamus, the thalamus, the cerebellum and the spinal cord. They are therefore particularly suited to governing the activation of the encephalon as a whole. Unless other regions of the brain inhibit them, some reticular neurons will send a continuous current of nerve impulses to the cerebral cortex, maintaining a state of wakefulness. The ascending reticular activating system is inhibited by the sleep centers situated in the hypothalamus, among other places.

It seems that the reticular formation is careful to sort the information which will be transmitted to the brain; it may be advisable for the osteopath to ensure that the information he gives the patient, through his hands, be 'selected' in order to avoid possible inhibition coming from other sensory pathways. This could suggest that when less information is received at any one time, the more the information received is unique, the more chance there is that this information becomes important. If other information were present at the same time, and if its intensity were greater than that proposed by the osteopath, the latter might not be taken into account.

The reticular formation also results in short-term synaptic facilitation in optical paths. This seems to mean that visual information is favored for some time. Since our work focuses on somatosensory information, perhaps it would be to our advantage to reduce the intensity of visual information to facilitate somatosensory information?

The thalamus

The thalamus is the major relay station for most sensory impulses which reach the primary sensory areas of the cerebral cortex from the spinal cord and brainstem. The signals passing through the thalamus are of two types:

–One type is rapidly transmitted action potentials which excite the cerebrum for only a few milliseconds. These originate from large neuronal cell bodies that lie throughout the brainstem reticular area. Their nerve endings release the neurotransmitter substance acetylcholine, which serves as an excitatory agent, lasting for only a few milliseconds before it is destroyed.

–The second type of excitatory signal originates from large numbers of small neurons spread throughout the brainstem reticular excitatory area. Again, most of these move toward the thalamus, but this time through small, slowly conducting fibers which synapse mainly in the intralaminar nuclei of the thalamus and in the reticular nuclei over the surface of the thalamus. From there, additional small fibers are distributed everywhere in the cerebral cortex. *The excitatory effect caused by this system of fibers can build up progressively for many seconds to a minute or more* (Hall and Guyton, 2011, p. 711), which suggests that its signals are especially important for controlling the long-term background excitability level of the brain. The level of activity of the excitatory area in the brainstem, and therefore the level of activity of the entire brain, is determined to a great extent by the number and type of sensory signals that enter the brain from the periphery.

And here's what is amazing. It has always been thought that nerve impulses travel at speeds calculated in milliseconds. *We learn here that in the brain, some information, going from the reticular formation to the cerebral cortex via the thalamus, can take up to a minute to make the journey.*

What is disturbing is that we are not sure what type of stimulation is required to activate these small interneurons which have very slow conduction, or what type of stimulation may inhibit the influx, or what kind of stimulation could prevent this journey.

What we do know is that these interneurons exist and that they are important for the longer term control of the background level of brain activity.

And if other, stronger, more intense information passes the filter of the reticular formation during this minute, is there not a risk of inhibiting the activity of these interneurons?

### Neurohormonal control of brain activity

One third of the brain's activating systems releases hormonal agents, excitatory or inhibitory neurotransmitters, into the substance of the brain. *These neurohormones often persist for minutes or hours and thereby provide long periods of control, rather than just instantaneous activation or inhibition* (Hall and Guyton, 2011, p. 712).

### An example of synergy between somatosensory stimulation, the central nervous system and the hormonal system

Stimulation of the cervix by the baby's head (somatosensory stimulation) during childbirth gives rise to nerve signals which pass through the hypothalamus to the posterior pituitary gland. Neurosecretory neurons going from the hypothalamus to the posterior pituitary gland release a neurohormone into the bloodstream: oxytocin, which in turn promotes more uterine contractions. Once labor has started, the oxytocin feedback mechanism (Fig. 1.10) helps create a cycle of ever more intense uterine contractions, which normally only stop when the baby is born.

*However, this never occurs without a pause.*

Indeed, the nerve receptors of the muscle fibers of the uterus must find a rest potential (relaxation after stretching) for another contraction to be effective, without however losing the level at which the fibers are stretched. Thus, when the uterine muscle receptors are adequate, the contraction stops, giving the receptors time to become more sensitive again, but not from their original stretch level: the fibers remain stretched. During the resting phase, the baby's head continues to press the stretched fibers until another contraction occurs with the arrival of more oxytocin released by the hypothalamus into the posterior pituitary gland and then by the posterior pituitary gland into the blood. This contraction must be stronger than the previous one in order to exceed the 'relative' resting potential obtained during the time of 'rest' between each contraction. This contraction pushes the baby onto the cervix, the fibers are stretched again, sending nerve impulses to the reticular formation, the thalamus and the hypothalamus, which in turn will

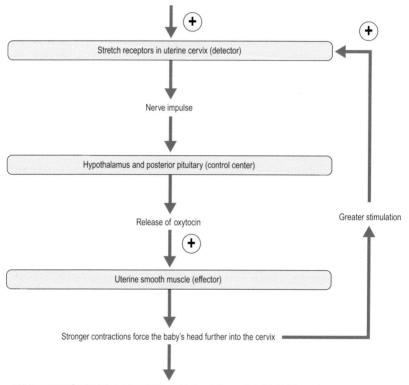

In labour, uterine contractions force the baby's head into the cervix

(+)

(+)

Stretch receptors in uterine cervix (detector)

Nerve impulse

Hypothalamus and posterior pituitary (control center)

Release of oxytocin

Greater stimulation

(+)

Uterine smooth muscle (effector)

Stronger contractions force the baby's head further into the cervix

Inhibition occurs after the delivery when uterine contractions no longer dilate (stretch) the cervix

**FIGURE 1.10**

Regulation of oxytocin secretion through a positive feedback mechanism. Reproduced with permission from Waugh and Grant, Anatomy and physiology in health and illness. p. 212. Elsevier 2010.

release oxytocin to a further contraction. And so on ... (Lehouelleur, 2015, p. 16).

Dr Michel Odent (2002), the French obstetrician who introduced the concept of hospital birthing rooms and birthing in pools, stresses some very interesting points that should be considered during labor.

Firstly, he emphasizes that we must better understand the factors that influence labor in order to make it as easy as possible. We must also better understand the hormonal process that occurs. These hormones are produced by the most primitive part of the brain – the hypothalamus and the pituitary gland. This part of the brain must work intensely to successfully complete the labor. *We must not disturb the woman giving birth with stimulations that would activate the cerebral cortex instead of the hypothalamus.* Lower the lights and avoid inappropriate discussions. Try not to watch the woman too much and understand her need for privacy. Reduce unnecessary nerve impulses as much as possible and avoid stimulating the neocortex to allow the nerve impulses required for a successful delivery. This is very interesting and is in the same line of thinking as the theory of 'minimal stimulation', i.e. only those which are necessary.

It must also be understood that the 'pause' between contractions is not without purpose. It allows receptors to recover their resting potential and gives time for the CNS to 'analyze' the situation and the hypothalamus to produce the exact amount of oxytocin needed for the next contraction. This is eloquent proof of the necessity of a pause during a self-regulating process.

Finally, another important point: *somesthesic stimulation affects the hypothalamus and the endocrine system.*

This example shows the importance of understanding neurological and endocrine mechanisms in order to act effectively on the body. See also Appendix II, for another example of research which shows the effect of extraocular light on the endocrine system, i.e. somatosensory stimulation in relation to the endocrine system.

### The important points

All information, whether transmitted by the spinothalamic tract or the posterior columns, will reach the reticular formation. From there, it is transmitted to other brain regions only if it passes through the filter of this system. In order to achieve this, stimuli must be more 'intense' or stronger or more unusual than other stimuli coming from the external or internal environment. But if this information were unique, if we reduced the impact of other external stimuli as much as possible, could we not increase the opportunity of it being 'heard' and passing through the filter?

Once 'selected' our stimulation will take one of two pathways through the thalamus: the fast lane or the slow lane. We cannot predict which pathway it will take. And if it took the slow lane, would it perhaps be beneficial to wait a minute, a little minute of security in order to avoid possible inhibition? Especially since this pathway appears to be important for the longer-term control of the background level of brain excitability.

We saw in the example of birth how somatosensory stimulation can activate (or favor) hormone production. We also know that the action of certain hormones can take time to be felt. The 'pause' between contractions allows the feedback mechanism to produce and release the right amount of oxytocin at the right time. Perhaps it would be beneficial to give a little time, as nature does, so that the brain prepares, develops and releases neurohormones or hypophysiotropic hormones, according to the situation or need, with an obvious intention of regulation.

### Notes

[1] Sir Charles Scott Sherrington was an English neurophysiologist, histologist, bacteriologist and pathologist. Sherrington and Edgar Adrian were awarded the Nobel Prize for Physiology or Medicine in 1932 for their work on the functions of neurons.

[2] 'Tact and touch are not synonymous. The sense of touch is concentrated in the hand; touch means to contact someone or something with your hand. It may be admitted that we also touch with the foot and with the lips. The tactile sensitivity is more extensive than that of touch. It extends not only over the surface of the skin but also at the orifices coated in mucous. It comprises the superficial sensitivity and deep sensitivity from our viscera and our musculoskeletal system'. (Lazorthes, 1986, p. 19).

[3] It is important to bear in mind that this thesis is related to the nervous system, not to other principles such as energy, fluidic exchanges and other exchanges which would be shared between the patient and the osteopath and whose existence would not call into question the physiological principles.

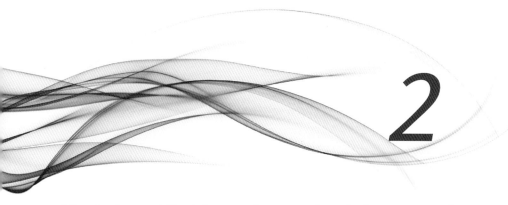

## Allostasis and limbic touch to maintain homeostasis

Homeostasis[1] refers to the processes that maintain the internal environment of the body within a narrow physiological range. It comes from the Greek roots *homeo*, meaning same, and *stasis*, meaning stable – remaining stable by staying the same. Homeostasis is involved particularly in the regulation of body temperature, the water/mineral balance, the precise regulation of blood volume, blood pressure, the acid-base equilibrium, the oxygen concentration and the glucose concentration. In other words, it is the system's capacity to maintain its functional balance in spite of external constraints. Its boundaries are very accurate and are expressed, for example, in the regulated settings of blood tests (blood glucose, creatinine, etc.). Blood pH should be between 7.35 and 7.45. These values cannot vary significantly without the body suffering serious consequences.

Consider temperature regulation. Biochemical reactions in many cells of the body are finely tuned to occur at about 37°C. A variation of more than a few degrees in either direction can be catastrophic. Temperature-sensitive cells in the hypothalamus detect variations in brain temperature and orchestrate the appropriate responses. (Bear, Connors and Paradiso, 2007, p. 484).

Different systems operate in much broader parameters in order to maintain homeostasis. This is what Professor Bruce McEwen, an expert in neuro-endocrinology, has described allostasis thus: "It comes from the Greek root *allo*, meaning variable, and it emphasises the point that allostatic systems help keep the body stable by being themselves able to change. Nowhere are these changes more dramatic than in the systems that comprise the stress responses" (McEwen, 2007). It is highly recommended that, as a therapist, you read McEwen's book *The End of Stress As We Know It* (McEwen, 2002).

Thus, homeostasis represents the regulatory processes which are essential to life and allostasis represents the systems which support these regulatory mechanisms.

### Allostasis

Allostatic systems help keep the body stable by being themselves able to change (McEwen, 2002, p. 6). It is the process by which the brain tries to promote short-term adaptation.

## 2

Take the example of an intense stress: a postman chased by a dog. The brain, which perceives the danger, links with the endocrine system which is primarily responsible for mobilizing the rest of the body and the immune system for internal defence. The main idea is to get the maximum amount of energy to the parts of the body that need it the most.

'Allostasis is often thought of as the "fight or flight" response because, taken to the extreme, it prepares for just those two eventualities.' But 'fight or flight' is allostasis with a sense of urgency. The purpose of allostasis is to help the organism remain stable in the face of any change and to provide enough energy to cope with any challenge – not just life-threatening ones.

'Take the simple fact of getting up in the morning. Some people consider it to be the first major trauma of the day. But, even for early birds, moving from sleep to wakefulness and from lying down to standing up makes demands on the body. To ensure sufficient energy to meet these demands, allostasis provides a higher level of stress hormones in the morning' (McEwen, 2002, p. 7). The hypothalamic–pituitary–adrenal (HPA) axis momentarily triggers to help us wake up and stand up. This response to 'stress' is part of normal physiology and is beneficial in the short term. This is allostasis.

### Allostatic load

The cumulative result of an allostatic state is allostatic load. It can be considered the result of the daily and seasonal routines which organisms carry out in order to obtain food and survive and obtain the extra energy needed to migrate, moult, breed, etc.

Allostatic load occurs when the activity and the levels of certain mediators (such as glucocorticoids which have a physiological role in all metabolisms) are destabilized, either too little or too much, in response to environmental changes or situations which represent a challenge. These challenges are, amongst other things, social and emotional relationships, temperature, disease, predators, pollution, poisoning, etc.

'The situations that ignite the stress response are ones for which neither fight nor flight is an option – working for an overbearing boss, for example, or caring for a family member who is seriously ill. In these situations the stress response cannot help speed us toward a resolution. And so, deprived from its natural result, the very system designed to protect us begins to cause wear and tear instead, and illness sets in' (McEwen, 2002, p. 7). The HPA axis is triggered and the higher rate of stress hormones risks becoming harmful and damaging if this condition persists.

Bruce McEwen identifies four ways in which the allostatic response can become allostatic load:

> Unremitting stress: This does not involve a malfunction per se; even the most finely tuned stress response in the healthiest of individuals can begin to cause damage if activated again and again over a long period. Chronic stress can cause illness, putting a strain on the heart, undermining the power of the immune system, and triggering processes that may lead to diabetes and other chronic illnesses.

> Inability to adjust: There are situations in which, though the stress itself is not lengthy or severe (a new job for example) the body responds in a way that is inappropriate.

> Incapacity to stop the stress response: Some people continue to have an allostatic response long after the stressful event has ended; there is evidence that genes may play a role.

> Too little is as bad as too much: When the stress response is insufficient, resulting in underproduction of the stress hormones, particularly cortisol, wear and tear can also result. Rheumatoid arthritis, allergies and asthma are some of the conditions linked with underproduction of cortisol.

> The first three scenarios involve long-term overexposure to adrenaline and cortisol, whether it's because the stress itself goes on too long, because the system cannot accommodate the fact that the situation should no longer be stressful or because the shutoff processes are not functioning. (McEwen, 2002, p. 56)

Other situations which can lead the body to a state of allostatic load are found in our way of life: lack of sleep, poor diet, lack or excess of exercise, diets, etc. The body can maintain an allostatic load for a limited time

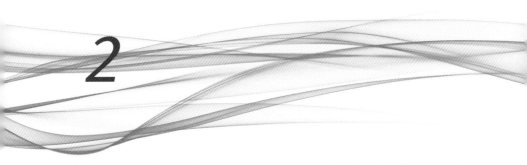

if it has enough stored energy to support and enable the homeostatic process. If the imbalance continues, allostatic overload symptoms occur.

## Allostatic overload

In their research 'The concept of allostasis in biology and biomedicine', Bruce McEwen and John C. Wingfield (2003) say that, within limits, the results of allostatic load are adaptive responses to seasonal and other demands. However, if one superimposes additional loads of unpredictable events in the environment such as disease, human disturbance, and social interactions, then allostatic load can increase dramatically.

They envision two distinctly different outcomes:

First, if energy demands exceed energy income, and what can be mobilized from stored energy, then 'Type 1 allostasis overload' occurs. For example, breeding birds use increasing food abundance in spring to raise young. If inclement weather then increases the cost of maintaining homeostasis in addition to the demands of breeding, and at the same time reduces food available to fuel this allostatic load, then negative energy balance results in loss of body mass and suppression of reproduction.

Second, 'Type 2 allostatic overload' occurs if energy demands are not exceeded and the organism continues to take in or store as much or even more energy that it needs. This may be a result of stress-related food consumption, choice of a fat-rich diet, or metabolic imbalances (prediabetic state) that favor fat deposition. There are other cumulative changes in other systems, e.g., neuronal remodeling or loss in hippocampus,[2] atherosclerotic plaques, left ventricular hypertrophy of the heart, glycosylated hemoglobin, and other proteins by advanced glysosylation end products as a measure of sustained hyperglycemia. High cholesterol with low HDL may also occur, and chronic pain and fatigue, e.g., in arthritis or psoriasis, associated with imbalance of immune mediators. (McEwen and Wingfield, 2003)

Thus, says Bruce McEwen, it may be possible to distinguish between allostatic load in the normal life cycle (incorporating unpredictable events in the environment) and allostatic overload that exceeds the capacity of the individual to cope.

According to Dr Giacomo Gastaldi and Dr Juan Ruiz, from the endocrinology faculty of Lausanne University, Switzerland, the new pandemic 'diabesity' (diabetes and obesity) is a consequence of allostatic overload (Gastaldi and Ruiz, 2009): 'Chronic stress in Western society can activate the autonomous, neuroendocrine and inflammatory/immunologic systems. Chronic exposure to stressors can indeed stimulate the hypothalamic–pituitary–adrenal axis and induce an imbalance between anabolic and catabolic hormones, responsible for an increase in visceral fat and of insulin resistance. These metabolic consequences can lead to prediabetes. Exposure to chronic stress results in allostatic load and its pathophysiologic consequences. The knowledge of these mechanisms and the related cardiovascular and metabolic risk, should influence our way of thinking about patient care. To decrease allostatic load, practitioners can rely on therapeutic relation. Therapeutic education is one of the skills that can be used to create therapeutic relation.'

For Bruce McEwen, management of chronic stress and allostatic load and overload should include:

### Brain-centered interventions

Because the brain is the central organ of the stress response, it is a primary target for interventions intended to reduce the burden of chronic stress, as defined by the concept of allostatic load and overload. In general, brain-centered interventions are very familiar in everyday life. They involve changing behavior and life-style, for example, by improving sleep quality and quantity, improving social support, and cultivating a positive outlook on life, along with maintaining a healthy diet, avoiding smoking, and engaging in regular, moderate physical activity.

### Pharmaceutical agents

It is important to note that there are many useful pharmaceutical agents, such as sleep medications, anxiolytics, beta blockers, and antidepressants, that counteract some of the problems associated with being stressed out. Likewise, drugs that reduce oxidative stress or inflammation, block cholesterol synthesis or absorption, and treat insulin resistance or chronic pain can help deal with the metabolic and neurological consequences of being 'stressed out.' All of these medications are valuable to some degree, yet each one has its side-effects and limitations.

**Physical activity**

A sedentary life-style is a major risk factor for many of the diseases of modern life including obesity, diabetes, cardiovascular disease, depression, and dementia, and recent studies have shown that moderate physical activity can be beneficial for the brain and cardiovascular and metabolic system.

**Social support**

Social support in the form of having regular social contacts with supportive friends or family or health professionals, who provide emotional support and provided useful information, has been shown to reduce the allostatic load score, which measures key physiological markers related to chronic stress and a potentially health damaging life-style. (McEwen, 2007)

## The sensual touch (or limbic touch)

Following research carried out by A.D. (Bud) Craig from the Barrow Neurological Institute in Phoenix, Arizona, I propose that manual therapy be added as an element which may be involved in the reduction of allostatic overload and in the regulation of homeostasis.

### *The basis*

Dr Craig is a functional neuroanatomist interested in the representation of feelings from the body, which affects theories of emotion and consciousness. His research focuses on sensory pathways and the role that certain neurons play in pain, temperature, itch, and other sensations related to the physiological condition of the body.

In his recent book *How do you feel? An Interoceptive Moment with your Neurobiological Self*, Dr Craig reminds us that Sir Charles Sherrington[3] classified senses into: teloreception (sensory inputs activated from a distance, i.e., vision and audition), proprioception (sensory inputs that relate to limb position), exteroception (sensory inputs activated from outside of the body), chemoreception (taste and smell) and interoception (sensations from the interior of the body, especially the viscera). He categorized nociception and thermoreception together with the sense of touch as aspects of exteroception, because he regarded all three as discriminative cutaneous sensations. Sherrington's codification underlies the conceptual organization of all modern neuroscience textbooks (Craig, 2015, p.3).

From these textbooks, Craig has noted that we find that almost all sensory information from the somatic segments of the body enters the spinal cord through the dorsal roots of the spinal nerves. From entry points into the cord and then to the brain, the sensory signals are carried through one of two alternative sensory pathways: the dorsal column for mechanoreceptors or the spinothalamic tract for pain and temperature sensations. These two systems come back together partially at the level of the thalamus and then are projected to the somatosensory (S1) cerebral cortex.

### The findings

Craig, as a graduate student, was very disturbed by what he called 'irritating incongruities' between pain and the somatosensory cortex. (We can follow in detail the development of the ideas in his book which, I believe, should first be studied thoroughly and then be kept as a bedside book by all manual therapists.) As he mentions on page 31 (Craig, 2015), it was already well known that neurosurgeons would not remove the postcentral cortex (an area of the cortex which includes the primary somatosensory cortex) in patients suffering from severe pain because experience had shown that it did not work. The same was true for temperature sensitivity; damage to the S1 produced no changes in thermal sensation, and no relief for patients who suffered from painful burning feelings produced by cool stimuli which are normally innocuous (cold allodynia). He also reminds us that Dr Penfield[4] never elicited a report of discrete pain sensation upon stimulation of the S1 cortex in conscious patients. Moreover, stimulation of S1 never produced a thermosensory feeling of cold or warmth on the skin.

The results of Dr Craig's research, which were published in 2000 (Craig et al., 2000 cited in Craig, 2015, p.35), firmly contradict the textbook

# 2

concept that temperature sensations are processed in somatosensory cortices S1 and S2, and they identify the terminus of the specific lamina I spinothalamic pathway in the dorsal posterior insular cortex. In addition, the results from this experiment reveal the interoceptive processing stream in the insular cortex and provide the first strong evidence that subjective feelings are engendered in the anterior insula.

## The afferent fibers

'The primary afferent A∂ and C-type fibers that are relayed by lamina I relate homeostatic information — that is, much more than simply 'pain and temperature' sensations — from all tissues. These fibers convey slow activity that is sensitive to changes in a wide variety of physiological conditions — not only temperature and mechanical stress, but also local metabolism (acidic pH, hypoxia, hypercapnia, hypoglycaemia, hypo-osmolarity and lactic acid), cell rupture (ATP and glutamate), cutaneous parasite penetration (histamine), mast cell activation (serotonin, bradykinin and eicosanoids), and immune and hormonal activity (cytokines and somatostatin).

'Particular observations emphasize that the category 'nociceptors,' while heuristically of enormous value, is actually a theoretical simplification of a larger reality. The primary afferent C-type fibers include the cutaneous C-fibers which are selectively and exquisitely sensitive to slow, weak mechanical stimuli that evoke sensual ('limbic') touch, as are neurons in lamina I and in the inner substantia gelatinosa' (Craig, 2002).

All small-diameter primary afferent sensory fibers from all tissue and organs of the body are going to land in lamina I interneurons, cross to the contralateral spinothalamic tract and reach the insular cortex where subjective feelings are engendered.

## The insula

In a conference held at the University of Linköping (Craig, 2009), Dr Craig explains that the insula is an island of tissue hidden deep inside the brain which is normally associated with visceral functions; it is the 'hidden lobe' of the brain. From the imaging studies available, it is shown that it does represent visceral sensations. Distention of the stomach will cause activation of the insula as well as the anterior cingulate.

The insula is activated not just by cooling, as was demonstrated in Dr Craig's studies (2002):

> '... but also by muscle pain, by laser-evoked C-fiber heat (laser pain to the skin), by deep visceral pain, as well as dynamic exercise, riding on a bicycle. They all activate homeostatic afferent input from A∂ and C-fibers from muscle whose main role is to guide the homeostatic nervous system, the autonomic nervous system, in its control of blood flow to muscle and skin. And that is what is happening within this part of the brain; it also represents itch and sensual touch because those are other aspects of the physiological condition of the body, which we can call 'interoception', that are important for cortical control of the physiological condition of the body.

> In fact, this now provides in the human brain a representation of feelings from the body. The primary encoding in the brain for a feeling sits right here, in posterior insula.' (Craig, 2009).

Amazingly enough, says Dr Craig, activation during anger and sadness and happiness and every human emotion that has been imaged in a scanner will cause activation in the same two places: in the insula and the anterior cingulate. This suggests that they are associated with autonomic function (Craig, 2009).

### The insular cortex and cingulate cortex

A.D. Craig's book is fascinating. On page 42, we can read: 'The combined lamina I + NTS homeostatic sensory pathways[5] to the dorsal posterior insular cortex represent the physiological condition of the entire contralateral body. It conveys highly resolved homeostatic sensory activity, the same sensory activity that drives the autonomic, neuroendocrine, and behavioral functions that support the process of homeostasis. The interoceptive cortex in the dorsal posterior insula of the human brain contains a primary sensory representation that underpins all of the affective feelings from the body, including cool, warm, pricking pain, burning pain, itch, visceral distension, muscle ache, hunger, thirst, 'air hunger,' sensual touch, and so on' (Craig, 2015).

*'The feelings from the body are each characterized by a distinct sensation that is inherently colored by a strong affect that is directly associated with a*

*2*

*motivation that drives behavioral responses needed to maintain the health
of the body; in other words, the affective feelings from the body occur concomitantly with motivations for homeostatic behavior'* (Craig, 2015).

For Dr Craig, these combinations can be viewed as *homeostatic
emotions.*

'All emotions can be characterized most simply as a feeling and a
concomitant motivation, and all subjectively experienced emotional
feelings are associated with conjoint activation of these two regions
in the brain: the insular cortex and the cingulate cortex. They are also
called limbic sensory cortex and limbic motor cortex respectively and
they can be thought of as representing the 'feeling' and the 'volitional
agency' that together form the fundamental neuroanatomical basis
for all human emotions' (Craig, 2015, p. 45).

### The sensual touch

'A particularly interesting sensory modality is limbic touch, also called
sensual touch. Limbic touch is an interoceptive modality. It serves
homeostasis at the level of the individual and also at the level of the
social community; it supports the health and well-being of the individual and the species' (Craig, 2015, p. 173).

Sensual touch is conveyed by small-diameter, unmyelinated C-tactile
sensory fibers with peripheral endings in the superficial dorsal horn
(lamina I). They innervate hairy skin all over the body; they are not
found in glabrous skin (e.g., the palm of the hand and the sole of the
foot). They are reported to be at least as numerous as C-nociceptors
or myelinated mechanoreceptors. The C-tactile sensory fibers are activated only by light brushing within a limited range of slow velocities
that are not fast enough to activate large-diameter cutaneous mechanoreceptors (Craig, 2015, p. 173).

They are responsible for the human sensation of affective touch
because they produce a feeling of 'pleasant' touch, that is, the feeling normally produced by close conspecific contact. They cause reflex
sympathetic activity, and they do not activate the somatosensory cortex but, rather, deactivate it and activate the dorsal posterior insular
cortex, like other C-fibers. They are sometimes called 'anti-nociceptors'

because they inhibit the central actions of nociceptive sensory fibers. Thus, there are homeostatic sensory fibers which signal safety, instead of danger (Craig, 2015, p. 109).

### Summary

Dr Craig proposes a new definition of the interoceptive sensitivity.

'Recentfindingsonthefunctionalanatomyofthelaminalspinothalamo-cortical system indicate that interoception should be redefined as the sense of the physiological condition of the entire body, not just the viscera. *This system is a homeostatic afferent pathway that conveys signals from small-diameter primary afferents that represent the physiological status of all tissues of the body.* It projects first to autonomic and homeostatic centers in the spinal cord and brainstem, *thereby providing the long-missing afferent complement of the efferent autonomic nervous system.* Together with afferent activity that is relayed by the nucleus of the solitary tract (NTS), it generates a direct thalamocortical representation of the state of the body that is crucial for temperature, pain, itch, sensual touch and other somatic feelings' (Craig, 2002, p. 1).

'The recognition that sensual touch is incorporated into the interoceptive system has strong implications for the neurobiological and health effects of conspecific contact' (Craig, 2002, p. 13).

*'The researches now seem to suggest that the anterior insula and anterior cingulate representation is a representation not only of how we feel, but of how we feel anything. That is to say our awareness, of ourselves, and our moment, and of others, and of environment: of human consciousness itself'* (Craig, 2009).

## Homeostasis in the hands of manual therapists

For the ultimate well-being of our patients, we must ask ourselves two questions:

1. Can a somato-insulo-sensory integration time influence the normalization of homeostasis?

2. Could the use of techniques which activate primary afferent C-fibers, by a kind of 'sensual' touch, influence homeostasis?

# 2

It seems that the answer for both questions is yes. For example, in one technique that I use and teach, we do one or two 'gentle moves' on some muscles or tendons, as if we were stretching them slowly, activating the type II afferent fibers of the spindle cells. We hold this stretch for a few seconds. Then we release and there is a pause of at least two minutes. During that time, the patient will often describe sensations in their body. Sometimes cold, sometimes heat, sometimes tingling or as if things were moving in their body. Some also talk about a different state of mind, as if they feel lighter but are, at the same time, sinking into the table. Some even describe a different awareness. For many years I have been teaching my students that when this happens strongly (the sensations can be very intense), we should wait until it calms down before touching the patient again, to avoid any kind of inhibitory process from other stimulations. The sensations can last five, 10 or even 15–20 minutes. In this technique, we know that the stimulations have reached the insular cortex because of the sensations that the patient is experiencing, which are 'homeostatic emotions'. However, we used the mechanoreceptors, and information from mechanoreceptors is going to reach the somatosensory cortex (S1), not the insula, unless the A$\partial$ primary afferent fibers were triggered from the deep pressure stimulation. In this case, there is a possible way to the insula. We also notice that the sensation can occur one or two minutes after the stimulation, which could signify that a waiting time is important, if not necessary, between mechanical stimulation and insular integration.

Another technique I use consists of very gentle 'line-drawings' on the skin. There is no pressure at all, no stretching of the skin; only a slow continuous touch, from the elbows to the tip of the fingers, from the knees to the tip of the toes and in the face, from the chin up to the vertex. The therapist uses both hands, 10 fingers to 'draw' the lines, passing a few times over each limb. Patients really appreciate this; they relax deeply and often the pain disappears, just by doing these 'line-drawings'. For a long time, I wondered what the physiology was behind this but after Dr Craig's discoveries, it is clear that we are affecting the primary afferent C-fibers and that this information is going to reach the insula which is at the heart of homeostasis.

It seems, according to research by Bruce McEwen and A.D. Craig, that there are ways to regulate homeostasis, for example, by becoming aware of allostatic load and reducing it, not only using pharmaceuticals, but by changes in lifestyle and possibly through direct intervention on the patient, especially in the form of limbic or sensual touch.

In addition to osteopathic techniques, already repeatedly recognized, and somato-insulo-sensory integration time which should take its rightful place, one of the ways of regulating homeostasis might indeed be through some specific manual therapy techniques, including the 'line-drawing' technique which I previously described and which is used by Niromathe (a manual therapy developed by Dr Raymond Branly) method practitioners. The lines drawn stimulate primary afferent C-fibers which, after passing through the lamina I, cross the spinal cord at the same level and reach the centers of homeostasis of the brainstem through the spinothalamic tract and continue their journey after another passage through the thalamus to the cortex and to the region of the anterior insular cortex. Remember that this region of the cortex is recognized, among others, as participating in interoceptive body consciousness. 'Activation in this area is correlated with subjective thermal sensation, with attention to pain, with subjective judgments of trust, disgust, anger, and happiness, and with sexual arousal, romantic love, and musical enjoyment' (Craig, 2003, p. 24).

The reading of fascinating books and scientific articles by Craig and McEwen suggests fields which have been little explored. Their findings and conclusions could be the basis for research to establish a more concrete, physiological link between manual therapy techniques which use C-tactile sensory fibers and the importance of a pause following stimulation involving mechanoreceptors and their effects on homeostasis.

Whilst awaiting work to be carried out in this field we already know that our action toward the patient will only be complete if we put it into perspective with the patient's allostatic charge or overload in order to reduce it and that the use of techniques such as sensual touch as well as therapeutic pauses is likely to strengthen the impact of our treatments on homeostasis. Thus, our response will be truly global, holistic.

Walter B. Cannon, who initiated the concept of homeostasis, would have said 'Vis medicatrix naturae'[6]

**2**

## Notes

[1.] The word homeostasis was first used in the mid-nineteenth century by a French scientist named Claude Bernard. He introduced the thinking that eventually led to the concept and science of stress. Bernard emphasized the body's need to maintain a constant state, what he called 'Le milieu intérieur'. Walter B. Cannon was an American physiologist, a professor at Harvard Medical School. He was one of the instigators of the concept of homeostasis after Claude Bernard.

[2.] 'The hippocampus is involved in remembering daily events and information, such as shopping lists, and names of people, places and things. The hippocampus is also important in the memory of context – the time and place of events, particularly those that have a strong emotional significance. Excessive levels of stress hormones interfere with the formation and retrieval of these memories, including those associated with context. This may add even more stress by blocking the informational input needed to decide that a situation is not a threat. Finally, the hippocampus is involved in the shutoff of the stress response. In sum, damage to this brain structure can both weaken our ability to perceive that something is not genuinely stressful and prevent the stress response from being shut off, thereby ratcheting up stress levels even higher' (McEwen, 2002, p. 62).

[3.] Sir Charles Sherrington received the Nobel Prize in Physiology or Medicine in 1932 for his studies of the motor system and the spinal cord.

[4.] Dr. Wilder Graves Penfield was a pioneering neurosurgeon at the Montreal Neurological Institute in the 1950s. He expanded brain surgery's methods and techniques, including mapping the functions of various regions of the brain such as the cortical homunculus.

[5.] Lamina I receives small-diameter sensory activity from regions innervated by sympathetic ANS fibers, and the NTS (nucleus of the solitary tract) receives small-diameter sensory activity from regions innervated by parasympathetic ANS fibers (Craig, 2015, p. 40).

[6.] The Hippocratic therapeutic approach was based on the healing power of nature; 'vis medicatrix naturae' in Latin. Walter B. Cannon resumed the concept: 'All that I have done thus far in reviewing the various protective and stabilizing devices of the body is to present a modern interpretation of the natural vis medicatrix' (Cross and Albury, 1987).

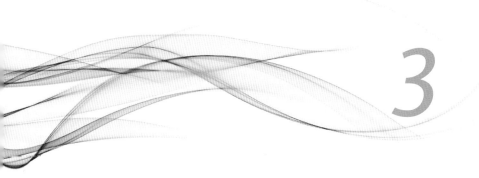

# 3

## Integration time in osteopathy

A general overview of some of the components of the nervous system, as it is currently known, was a necessary prerequisite for understanding pauses that exist in osteopathy and other manual therapies.

Pauses are indeed part of osteopathy, without them necessarily being named as such. They exist mainly in cranial osteopathy and fluidic osteopathy techniques. The latter detects structural and fluidic (dynamic) dysfunctions of the body and teaches the body how to correct itself and gradually regain its balance. The pause is, however, not as obvious in structural techniques (spinal and peripheral joint manipulation) or during the application of techniques such as osteopathic articulation, soft tissue manipulation, myofascial release or visceral manipulation during which the manipulations follow one after another. Or, if they are present, it is because the therapist has chosen to include them, not because he has been taught to do so. Based on our current conception, it is perhaps here that we should think about adding somato-insulo-sensory integration time.

Now let's look at osteopathy through the eyes of well-known osteopaths such as Sutherland, Becker, Still, Jealous, Upledger, Tricot, Duval, Sergueef and Fernandez, and try to identify times when osteopaths use pauses.

### Fluctuation of the cerebrospinal fluid (CSF)

'The CSF occupies a closed space divided into two distinct compartments: a deep ventricular space, and another, superficial, subarachnoid space. These two compartments are connected at the 4th ventricle', says Lazorthes (1973, p. 484).

The volume of the cavity containing the entire encephalon and the spinal cord is approximately 1600 ml. The volume of CSF is constant, at an average of 140 ml, 25 ml of which is in the ventricles and the remaining 115 ml in the subarachnoid spaces and cisterns (see also studies on the variation of the volume of the CSF with aging (Kohn et al., 1991). All of these cavities are connected and the pressure of the liquid is regulated to remain at a constant level.

CSF comes from blood plasma; however, it is produced by secretion, not by filtration. Qualitatively, it has the same composition as blood; all the substances that are found in CSF are also found in blood. There are, however, some important quantitative differences: in particular, CSF contains little protein, fewer sugars and a greater concentration of chlorides. CSF is therefore not simply a plasma filtrate.

'CSF is formed at a rate of about 500 ml each day, which is three to four times as much as the total volume of fluid of the entire CSF system. About two thirds or more of this fluid originates as secretion from the choroid plexuses in the four ventricles, mainly in the two lateral ventricles. Additional small amounts of fluid are secreted by the ependymal surfaces of all the ventricles and by the arachnoidal membranes. A small amount comes from the brain itself through the perivascular spaces that surround the blood vessels passing through the brain' (Hall and Guyton, 2011, p. 746).

The CSF formed in the lateral ventricles and the 3rd ventricle runs through the aqueduct of Sylvius to the 4th ventricle, where the quantity of liquid formed is even greater. It then runs through the small ducts of Luschka and the foramen of Magendie (the median aperture) into the large cistern, a large liquid-filled space behind the bulb and underneath the cerebellum. It finally reaches the subarachnoid spaces, which are a prolongation of the large cistern surrounding the brain and spinal cord. Almost all the liquid will flow toward the brain through this space. From the subarachnoid spaces, the liquid circulates up to the arachnoid villi that project onto the sagittal venous sinus and other sinuses. It finally rejoins the venous blood through the surfaces of these villi. Reabsorption may also take place in the vertebral and intervertebral venous plexus as well as in the lymphatic vessels. 'Lymphatic resorption through perineural spaces: subarachnoid injection of Indian ink allows grains to be found in the cranial nerve sheaths, and even as far as the lymph nodes. During lipiodolized[1] spinal exploration, the contrasting substance can diffuse very slowly along the spinal nerve roots and trunk' (Lazorthes, 1973, p. 494).

(Lipiodolization is the injection of lipiodol or poppyseed oil for use as a radio-opaque contrast agent to outline structures in radiological investigations.)

According to Dr Lazorthes, it cannot be denied that the CSF circulates from its source to the areas of reabsorption. CSF is not stagnant, he says. It is more of a slow fluctuation, a mass displacement, rather than real circulation. He adds that there are no large streams of liquid, but rather eddies resulting from respiration, changes in the volume of the brain, alterations caused by effort, coughing and pressure variations due to arterial beats.

Kamina (2008, p. 415) adds that the circulation of CSF is enabled by the pulsations of the choroidal arteries, the beating of the ependymocytes' cilia, but it is also due to the fact that venous pressure is low. He would tend to agree with Dr Lazorthes: In his opinion, although the reabsorption of CSF is essentially venous, it can also take place in the lymphatic system and in the nasal membranes through the intermediary of the olfactory nerves.

Osteopathy provides complementary notions. Adah S. Sutherland tells us, concerning the first experiment on the compression of the 4th ventricle, that William Sutherland felt 'a remarkable movement of fluid, up and down the spinal column, throughout the ventricles, and surrounding the brain. [...] He consulted Webster's Dictionary. Fluctuation was defined as 'the movement of fluid contained in a natural or artificial cavity'.[...] Furthermore, palpation was possible and fluctuation detectable by the sensitive use of thinking-seeing-feeling-knowing fingers' (Sutherland, 1962, pp. 40–41). He considered that he was entitled to demonstrate that, just as it is possible to observe the rhythm of blood flow in the beat of a pulse, it is possible to observe the rhythmic fluctuation of the CSF through the sense of touch. The term 'fluctuate' is used here to describe a wave-like motion which repeatedly rises and falls. For example, if water is placed in a flat plastic bag and pressure is applied to different areas of the bag, the water will fluctuate with successive rising and falling motions similar to waves. With this image in mind, in the circulation of CSF, the movement of the intracranial membranes produces pressure which animates the liquid giving successive rising and falling waves. He then refined this notion of 'waves' into a 'tide' in order to express a more powerful meaning: 'The movement of the tide is the movement of that body of water, the ocean, that constant body of water. See that potency in the tide; more power, more potency in that tide than there is in the waves that come dashing upon the shore.' (Sutherland, 1990).

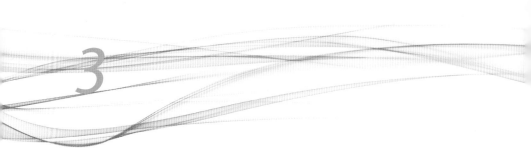

Thus, in considering Dr Sutherland's work, we do not yet speak of the rhythm of CSF per se, but rather of a rhythmic fluctuation which varies opportunistically according to circumstance.

Dr Rollin Becker DO perceived two types of 'tide' or rhythmic fluctuation. The first 'tide' occurs eight or 12 times per minute. The osteopath can alter it using a number of techniques. The other tide, 'the great tide' occurs around six times every 10 minutes. It arises spontaneously, grows slowly and takes around 45 seconds to develop completely. This is followed by a short pause, after which the tide retreats, taking the same amount of time as it took to rise. After another pause it begins to rise again, and so on. The practitioner can feel a progressive build-up of fluid throughout the body, an expansion and a sensation of plenitude in each cell, space and vessel. Once it has reached its peak, the wave gradually retreats. Dr Becker considered this a physiological process of general self-regulation:

*'In order to have a tide, there has to be an incoming tide, a pause-rest point, an outgoing tide, a pause-rest point, and so on. At the fulcrum point — at the point where the tide changes from one direction to the other — is the point at which the Breath of Life interchanges with the cerebrospinal fluid'* (Becker, 2001, p. 6).

Let us return to the phenomenon of the reabsorption of CSF. It is unsettling to note that, in addition to setting out the foundations of the primary respiratory mechanism (PRM) and defining the physiological actions of the CSF, according to Alain Croibier DO, Sutherland suggested that when this liquid moves throughout the body like a tide, it travels through the microtubules of the fascia (Croibier, 2005, p. 17).

Would the gel inside the polyhedral fibrillar armature that Dr Guimberteau speaks of (see Appendix III) be CSF which, pushed by Becker's great tide, is distributed throughout the body by Dr Sutherland's fascia microtubules, into Dr Lazorthes' perineural junctions?[1] How could it be transported throughout the body? Dr Guimberteau's research may provide a possible solution by explaining how the fibrils' ability to fuse, split, slide, dilacerate and rearrange themselves allows them to share their contents with their neighboring fibrils. The distribution of CSF could perhaps be partially ensured, the vehicle being the collagen fiber which is thought to be the organizational framework of the living structure. These assumptions are not thus expressed by Dr Guimberteau and are pure speculation on our part. Other indications (see Appendix IV) lead us to believe that there is a direct link between the CSF and collagen fibers of the fascia.

The intrinsic rhythm of CSF has not been clearly identified; it is a fluctuating circulatory movement induced originally at the production stage. We must, however, go further and understand the second step necessary in the establishment of this rhythm: the development of the primary respiratory mechanism.

## The primary respiratory mechanism (PRM)

According to William Sutherland, as an involuntary mechanism, the primary respiratory mechanism includes the highest known element: the cerebrospinal fluid that contains the invisible Breath of Life:

> The primary mechanism consists of the fluctuation of the cerebrospinal fluid within and around the brain and spinal cord, fundamentally. The motility of the brain and spinal cord, the mobility of the cranial bones and the sacrum between the ilia, and the intracranial and intraspinal membranes, functioning as reciprocal tension agencies between poles or articular attachment, are also included. (Sutherland, 1998, p.216)

The cranial joints have involuntary mobility and do not make use of an intermediary muscular mechanism although they are influenced externally by attachments and the movements of all musculoskeletal chains of the body connected to external cranial fascia. Internally, however, they possess a special intracranial membrane tissue that serves not only as an intermediary, but also as a reciprocal tension agent which limits normal joint mobility. This function is performed by the falx cerebri and the tentorium cerebelli, which can lead to movement in the joints while simultaneously regulating or limiting normal joint mobility. While respiration occurs, during the inspiration phase, the reciprocal tension membrane allows the crista galli to drop down while pulling the clinoid processes of the sphenoid bone upward, the petrous pyramids of the temporal bones upward and the occiput forward. During the expiration phase, the inverse of these movements occurs. 'The membranes are assisted by the reciprocal tensions of the external musculoskeletal chains, whose tensions vary during breathing, to make the skull open like a flower' (Robitaille, 2009).

During his experiments on the 4th ventricle, Sutherland not only felt the fluctuation of the CSF. He exclaimed to his wife, Adah: 'Believe or not, there also was a movement of my sacrum!' (Sutherland, 1962, p. 40). This was the 'Eureka!' moment for osteopathy, or at the very least, the beginning of craniosacral osteopathy: This mechanism works in such a way that the dura mater lifts the sacrum around its axis into a position of respiratory flexion, lifting the base up and the apex forward. This is the movement the sacrum makes between the ilia.

Another element enters into the orchestra of the intrinsic movement of the brain and the spinal cord. Its inherent motility, similar to that of the jellyfish, can be observed during surgery. During the inspiration phase, the cerebral hemispheres balance upwards like the wings of a bird; the 3rd ventricle dilates and lifts the body of the hypophysis (pituitary gland), which is firmly attached by the dural membranes to the sella turcica. This lifting of the sella turcica causes the anterior extremity of the sphenoid bone to tilt downwards. At the same time, the spinal cord is pulled upwards. An inverse movement occurs during expiration.

But the key to how the PRM works is, without a doubt, the circulation of cerebrospinal fluid: the full significance of the CSF is brought to light here. 'The arterial stream *is* supreme *but* the cerebrospinal fluid is in command', Sutherland would say (Sutherland, 1998, p. 231). The tension of the intracranial and intraspinal membranes, acting as a brake on the membranes during respiration, initiates the fluctuation of the cerebrospinal fluid.

'All musculo-fascial chains seem also to be involved. The PRM is a movement which is integrated throughout the whole body.'

'The movement of the PRM is constant, rhythmic; it can vary in its rising and falling, and even demonstrates plateaus; it functions as a cycle. The movement of each bone is synchronized with all the others and with the movement of the CSF, from the neural axis to the meninges and, where possible, through the tension frames of the human body, thus constituting a real physiological unit' (Robitaille, 2009).

So, like the conductor of an orchestra, the osteopath can create harmony with his hands by normalizing the body's profound rhythm.

## The 'still point'

There are many typical signs that indicate the conclusion of a release of the energy charge retained in the tissue (Tricot, 2005, p. 116), whether it be mechanical or somato-emotional. The first, the one that is of interest here, is the diminishment of a releasing process which progressively slows down until it stops at a 'still point.' This phrase, 'still point,' used by cranial osteopaths, can be understood as a moment of immobility. There are two types:

> The physiological 'still point' which habitually occurs in all alternative phenomena. Each period of time taken by the phenomenon is separated by an instant during which the phenomenon moving in one direction stops before changing direction. At this time, energy potential can build before manifesting itself once again in movement.

> The resolution 'still point' corresponds to the moment of resolution in a retention zone; the moment when the structure, having released retained energy, is in a state of waiting, just before opening the lines of communication. This immobility can last some time: It is essential that the practitioner be mindful of this and wait.' (Tricot, 2005, p. 308)

### What happens during the 'still point'?

Searching for the 'still point' is not necessarily the goal of osteopathic treatments. 'A still point is a physiologic balancing act that the body physiology of any patient is going through. It can occur anytime, anywhere, anyhow. It probably occurs spontaneously in patients during a good night's sleep or something like that. It is the body's attempt to release itself to a total motile mechanism. In a treatment, it is an observable event that the physician can recognize as having taken place within the body physiology but not one that he deliberately is seeking nor is he trying to evaluate it. The fact that it does take place indicates that the body physiology chooses to use it' (Becker, 2006, p. 69).

The 'still point' can also be induced by the therapist to facilitate the release of tension in the membranes around the brain and the spinal cord. A delicate and momentary interruption of the flow of liquids temporarily congests the system. Once the tissue is relaxed and the fluids begin to circulate again, they 'purge' the system, and in doing so lightly stretch the membranes which encourages the relaxation of restrictions and adhesions in the tissue. As well as increasing blood circulation toward the brain, this method has therapeutic effects on the central nervous system and the body as a whole, soothing headaches and muscle pain, reducing stress, providing a deep sense of relaxation and a general sense of well-being.

This is what Sutherland had to say about it:

> Bring the fluctuation of the cerebrospinal fluid down to its rhythmic balance where all the fluids have that immediate interchange between the cerebrospinal fluid and the blood. Do you get the picture? An interchange from the chemicals in the blood with those in the cerebrospinal fluid (Sutherland, 1998, p. 342).

Magoun explains:

> The intent of this technic (compression of the fourth ventricle) is to slow down fluctuation to a brief, rhythmic sequence most favorable for interchange throughout the fluids of the body. There is also a relaxation of secondary lesions in the spine. The evidence is consistent that with this technic there is an intensified interchange between all the fluids of the body. The reaction is unmistakably systemic, resembling the effect of a "lymphatic pump". The short, rhythmic strokes of the diaphragm act on the cisterna chyli, the thoracic duct and all the fascias of the body. With the continuity of fluids and of tissues the entire body can be influenced by this one action (Magoun, 1976, p. 110).

Osteopaths often describe a release of heat. These sensations signal that a local or overall recalibration has taken place and that functional activities have been improved. Ultimately, the osteopath ensures that order is well established and that 'Nature will do the rest' (Gravett, 1948, citation number 23).

## Pierre Tricot DO: energy saturation and refusal

### *Energy saturation*

Pierre Tricot DO asked himself how and why energy could be stored in corporal structures. The recognized field of basic paramedical study did not provide him with any answers. He found a solution to the question in the example of whiplash.

'When a person has a seat belt on, the head is the most mobile part of the body. The violence of the shock subjects the body to particularly brutal movements which are transmitted by the dura mater to the sacrum where the arrival of an intense flux produces the phenomenon of whiplash […]. With whiplash, an energy charge is transmitted to all corporal structures. All of these structures together, the fascia included, take on the charge and send it throughout the body, where it is dissipated through movement. When the tissue structures do not manage to dissipate the energy produced and if there is no rupture, some of it seems to be retained. There is a saturation of energy wherever a tissue structure does not transmit and dissipate the kinetic energy it has received' (Tricot, 2005, p. 94). This phenomenon is Tricot's energy saturation.

In the concept of inertia there is a relationship between two fundamental elements: energy and time. The energy/time relationship determines whether the living structure will absorb or dissipate the energy charge received. The same charge transmitted over a longer period of time would not provoke the same problems: the corporal structures would have enough time to dissipate it.

To understand the tissue reaction to kinetic energy, Tricot suggested imagining an immobile boat on water. If there is enough energy to move it forward, we can choose to transmit this energy in one of two ways. In the first method, we transmit an energy charge over a very short time, resulting in an intense but brief force. In this case, the boat will not advance far, because, since its inertia in the water was not accounted for, it behaves as though fixed to it, the greater part of the energy transmitted having been deflected. In the second method, the energy charge is spread out over a long period of time. The force created is less intense but persistent, and the boat moves forward easily.

**3**

The time needed to mobilize a body depends on its mass and the medium through which it is moving. We could have the audacity to make a parabolic analogy. 'The Archimedes principle applied along the horizontal axis is in this case related to the force of inertia rather than the gravitational force' (Racano, 2014).

'More time is needed to overcome the inertia of a body in water than a body in the air. Knowing that at least 65% of the human body is made up of water we can imagine that, when an external solicitation demands a response from tissue, a certain amount of time is required ...' (Tricot, 2005, p. 95) ... and this same body will also need time to 'dissipate' the energy induced by the therapist or to 'integrate' information.

## Refusal

Pierre Tricot describes a method of validating the tissue's resistance to release. By reinforcing its resistance, the practitioner can assist in a release of tension. Applying his intention and verbally or mentally encouraging the zone in its resistance, he aggravates the lesion. Validating the conscience of the tissue in its resistance – acknowledging that, at the moment it occurred, it was a reasonable way of ensuring the survival of the individual – tends to open the lines of communication. According to Pierre Tricot, the conscience senses validation and invalidation. This process works subtly with the conscience's propensity to protect itself through refusal. It will tend to refuse whatever is asked of it. If one works with its refusal, however, it will not be able to keep it up, and the lines of communication will be re-opened. When the practitioner stimulates the structure and encourages its refusal, it sinks deeper into its retention, releasing energy until it returns to a neutral point, a still point, and then expands slightly.

Although Pierre Tricot does not talk about a 'pause' as such, it seems clear that he considers it important to 'slow down, slow down, slow down as it is when the tissue very slowly reaches its space/time maximum inertia that release occurs' (Tricot, 2009).

The lapse of time when the therapist waits and leaves the tissue (or body or CNS) to react is a somato-insulo-sensory integration time. That is to say, for the therapist himself, it is not a pause, as he/she must remain highly vigilant in order to feel the release. For the patient, it is at the afferent level that the pause occurs (hence the name somato-insulo-sensory integration time). There is no pause in the patient's CNS. On the contrary, it is at this moment that the body reacts the most; that it can react, whilst no other afferent 'disturbs' the process implemented by the osteopath.

## Nicette Sergueef DO: the Traube–Hering wave – an accidental pause

'The primary respiratory mechanism (PRM) shown by a cranial rhythmic impulse (CRI), a fundamental concept in cranial osteopathy, and the Traube–Hering–Meyer (THM) oscillation are strikingly similar. For this reason, a protocol was developed in order to measure simultaneously the two phenomena. Statistical comparisons demonstrated that the CRI is palpable concomitantly with the low frequency variations of the THM oscillation' (Sergueef, Nelson and Glonek, 2001).

Seen in arterial pressure, the rate of blood flow and heart rate, the Traube–Hering oscillation has a frequency of six to 10 cycles per minute. First described by Traube and Hering at the end of the nineteenth century, its frequency seems similar to that of the cranial rhythmic impulse (CRI). Laser Doppler flowmetry readings have shown a correlation between the Traube–Hering–Mayer oscillation in the blood circulation and the CRI.

On two separate occasions, during their work with the Transonic Laser Doppler Monitor BLF21 Series, they had the opportunity to observe marked changes in the amplitude of the TH wave before and after manipulative treatment. These significant differences are worth mentioning.

Initially, the two subjects presented low amplitude TH wave fluctuations in the blood flow rate.

Subject 1 is a 55-year-old male. Subject 2 is a 25-year-old female. Neither presented any physical or medical condition requiring medication. The cranial exam revealed a diminished cranial rhythmic impulse (CRI), particularly in Subject 1.

The treatment for Subject 1, which lasted approximately 10 minutes, consisted of normalization of the craniocervical junction and of the anterior–posterior movement in the cranium. The treatment for Subject 2, which lasted approximately 15 minutes, consisted of normalization of the craniocervical junction and of the cranial base.

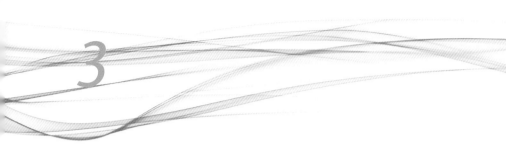

**FIGURE 3.1**
Subject 1 – before treatment

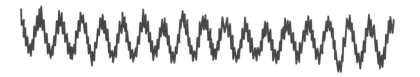

**FIGURE 3.2**
Subject 2 – before treatment

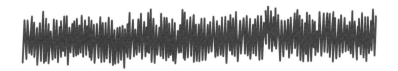

**FIGURE 3.3**
Subject 1 – after treatment

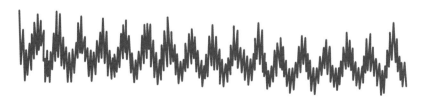

**FIGURE 3.4**
Subject 2 – after treatment

Figures 3.1–3.4 are the laser Doppler monitor readings of the rate of blood flow for the two individuals before and after treatment. Each of these represents approximately three minutes of continuous recording. They have not been modified, and were recorded at 20-minute intervals. The high frequency oscillation observed in the four recordings is the variation in the blood-flow rate with the cardiac systoles and cardiac diastoles. The low-frequency oscillation, absent in the pretreatment recordings and present in the two post-treatment recordings, is the TH oscillation.

From our point of view, there is one variable which was not evaluated and which could, along with the treatment received, have influenced the results: the waiting time between the end of the treatment and the second reading. If 20 minutes passed between each three-minute series of readings and the treatment lasted between 10 and 15 minutes, there would be a 5- to 10-minute pause before the next reading (Fig. 3.5).

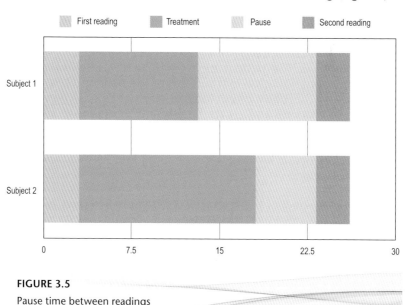

**FIGURE 3.5**

Pause time between readings

Research such as that carried out by Nicette Sergueef and colleagues could be a good starting point for further study with the aim of assessing the importance of a pause between the two techniques.

For example a reading could be taken straight after treatment and another 10 minutes later.

## Rollin Becker DO: the moment of calm

The osteopath, Rollin Becker used the expression 'pause' or 'rest.' In 'Techniques to Achieve Balance in Physiological Functioning in Anatomicophysiological Mechanisms' he explains the techniques he used to normalize the physiological functions of the anatomicophysiological mechanisms (Becker, 2001, p. 77).

Here, in summary, is how he explains his techniques:

> Basically, the physician is trained in anatomy, physiology, pathology and all other allied sciences to clinically evaluate health and to do something for the patient with medicine, surgery or other modalities; to diagnose and treat trauma and disease. Rhythmic balanced interchange techniques require that the physician goes another step deeper into the understanding of the body physiology[2] of the patient by working with and through the anatomicophysiological mechanisms of the patient, utilizing the potency of the body physiology of the patient as the motive power to evaluate and create health and to diagnose and correct existing trauma and disease.' (Becker, 2001, p. 78)

These techniques, in his view, are real methods of self-regulation and auto-normalization.

> 'The primary goal of the resources of body physiology is to create health for the individual. The tendency of body physiology is always toward health. When trauma or disease is added to body physiology, it resists or adapts to the limitations imposed upon it and continues to seek health in anatomicophysiological functioning. It is the intelligent use of rhythmic balanced interchange techniques in addition to medical and/or surgical intervention if necessary, that will give the most efficient care to the body physiology of the patient in its time of need. The capacity of body physiology to heal itself cannot be overestimated. (Becker, 2001, p. 82)

Along with medical intervention, rhythmic balanced interchange techniques allow the physiology of the body to use its own resources to evaluate and normalize itself after a trauma or when under the effects of disease.

Indeed, 'when the harmful effects of trauma or illness have exceeded the self-regulation capacity of a functional unit of the body, it is necessary to provide a stable fulcrum for this functional unit so that it can, once again, regain its ability to self-assess and self-regulate' (Robitaille, 2009).

Table 3.1 summarizes the therapist's actions and the objective of each action:

| The therapist's action | The therapist's conscious attention and tactile sensitivity allows him to: |
|---|---|
| The therapist refers to the patient's history to select the key area | Evaluate the health of the patient's tissues. How healthy is he/she? |
| The therapist places his hands on the key area and applies moderate, controlled pressure on the implicated tissue. <br>– The therapist establishes a fulcrum within the physiology of the patient's body. <br>– The physiology of the patient's body begins to develop a rhythmic activity of exchange and balance in the implicated tissue. The therapist can feel this | Evaluate the tone and quality of the tissue in the zone of action, the site of the trauma or of the disease and determine how the tissue there is implicated |
| The therapist, using his hands and sense of touch, becomes an integral part of the process and can feel the moment when the tissue is in a state of equilibrium | Evaluate the reaction time of the multiple layers of the fascia, membranes and ligaments. Draw the tissue towards a rhythmic equilibrium |
| During this 'pause', the therapist's hands remain in contact with the key area until he feels a change in the tissue. He will feel, after a period of inaction, a release in the zone that will lead to more harmonious functioning in the physiology of the body | Evaluate the equilibrium obtained in the tissue in the zone of action |

**Table 3.1**

Summary of the therapist's actions and objectives

'It may take a few minutes to direct the first key area through its treatment cycle, but once the physiology of the body has responded, the other key areas will react relatively quickly.' wrote Jacques Andreva Duval (2008, p. 68), one of Rollin Becker's students. Becker himself was taught by William G. Sutherland who had been taught by Andrew T. Still.

The practitioner must pause until the body signals that it has completed its cycle. In his book, *Techniques ostéopathiques d'équilibre et d'échanges réciproques*, Jacques Andreva Duval continues:

> We can suggest that the time needed to complete a treatment cycle, from the moment of contact to the return to the equilibrium point and beyond, varies according to the quality of the tone of the tissue being treated. The strength of healthy tissue makes it easy to work with: it will respond relatively quickly. Tissue affected by trauma or disease is locally fatigued. In this case it may take more time for the equilibrium point to be felt; or, if the tissue is weak, there may be quick but limited improvement that same day. The next treatment may have an acutely powerful effect, with less local fatigue and a greater response to the treatment cycle.

> Tissue affected by a generalized or chronic disease usually responds extremely slowly and weakly. Similarly, the response of tissue affected by medication, tranquilizers in particular, is often delayed and uncertain. In all cases, regardless of the condition being treated, the patient's physiology will provide the maximum response possible and it will be the most effective response it can offer.

Once the tissue has normalized, **the therapist waits and observes until, after a period of inaction, he feels a release in the treated zone**.

'This wait requires a fulcrum to be maintained so that that the body is informed of the change. It then self-assesses and triggers a rebalancing around this new state: it is necessary and essential that the therapist not only waits, but also observes' (Robitaille, 2009).

Rollin Becker also explains that the patient's self-regulation mechanisms will fairly rapidly initiate a response, often in the form of a reflex arch. But it will also initiate responses from the CNS and the ANS that can take many seconds or even minutes. His words:

The patient's body mechanism initiates a response – the simple reflex arc, which is relatively quick – into the cord and out again. But it also initiates the responses of the central and autonomic nervous systems that go to the brain, participate in all the sensory interchange in the brain, and produce an outflow that finds its way back down through all these tissues. This occurs more slowly, taking a matter of seconds or minutes.

He says that the therapist must maintain the fulcrum with the patient in order to feel the responses coming from the nervous system. When this mechanism is initiated, it tends to need to 'play out' in order to return to its route toward equilibrium and a point of rest, a 'still point' (Becker, 2001, p. 117).

## Daniel Fernandez DO: a somato-sensory integration time?

Daniel Fernandez DO is also a physiotherapist who practices and teaches osteopathy. The effectiveness of osteopathy's therapeutic movements was observed in ultrasounds carried out by Fernandez with electro-radiologist, Dr Annette Lecine. Their studies did not examine integration time, but Fernandez mentions pauses at least three times in his book (Fernandez and Lecine, 1988).

He mentions one on page 228 in his description of an emotional release technique that works through the treatment of overall movement:

This technique is reminiscent of the compression of the 4th ventricle that can be followed as it tightens, keeping it from returning to its original state until a healing 'still point' is obtained. The principle is the same: *You must recognize the pauses in the subject's body and wait without moving (maintain the fulcrum and observe). When the rhythm returns, the movement is followed again, through its largest axis, and so on, until emotional relaxation is obtained.* [...] When the 'still point' arises, we let it express itself without moving; as soon as the rhythm returns, we once again follow the movement along its larger axis, keeping it from returning to its point of departure.

More surprisingly, on page 172, we read in the description of a releasing technique used for the psoas:

> The psoas can be tight either in its entirety or only the superior or the inferior part. We do not distinguish one arch from another. Our fingers search for the tightest area superiorly or inferiorly. We maintain light pressure which remains slightly above the pain threshold, and ask the subject to breathe regularly, calmly, with eyes closed, without changing position. After a few minutes the psoas relaxes under our fingers, and the tension harmonizes with the opposite side. *The subject should rest for a few minutes in the same position before moving.*

Fernandez does not offer any explanation for this pause here, nor later on page 291 when, discussing a gallbladder treatment, he affirms that 'the gallbladder treatment really ends while waiting for the zone to reheat under the palm of your hand, you can then let your patient rest before the next treatment.

Despite not explaining the reason for this pause, Fernandez sensed its importance as he took the trouble to note it.

## John E. Upledger DO: the resting point

John E. Upledger DO, FAAO was the director of the Upledger Institute in West Palm Beach, Florida. As Professor of Biomechanics at the College of Osteopathic Medicine, Michigan State University, he conducted scientific work and clinical research which constitute the foundations of craniosacral therapy. He used 'modification of craniosacral rhythm techniques.' The aim of these techniques is to introduce new mobility to the craniosacral system by helping it find new passages. This involves following the craniosacral movement in its most natural expression until it reaches its maximum amplitude or its physiological limit and resisting its return.

With each cycle, the therapist captures the movement as it is renewed, until he feels the onset of the resting point through rough irregularities in the craniosacral mobility: shivers, pulsations or oscillations, for example. The therapist continues to resist the return of the mobility to the neutral positions and inevitably, activity in the craniosacral system ceases. This is the resting point.

*During this resting point, complete release occurs. Pain disappears and the somatic dysfunction can be spontaneously corrected. Respiration is liberated and all muscular tension seems to disappear. The resting point can last anywhere from a few seconds to a few minutes.* The craniosacral system then returns to its state of mobility, usually with improved symmetry and greater amplitude. This technique of inducing a resting point can be used on any point on the body.

## James Jealous DO: the neutral point

Dr Jealous studied with Dr Becker. He continued and furthered the research started by Becker and Sutherland. His concept of the neutral point is completely original. One day when they were working together, Dr Becker told him that that he was beginning the treatment too soon and that he should wait until the patient accepted that the primary respiratory mechanism was directing the body, not the ego. According to Dr Becker, as long as the ego is in control of the system, the disease cannot be cured.

Dr Jealous then understood the necessity of waiting for that moment when the body, in all its manifestations, becomes completely whole.

He explains how, at the start of a treatment, one must resist the urge to follow the tissue, induce a movement and begin a therapeutic process:

> All the movements the osteopath senses originate in the central nervous system and have the purpose of bringing equilibrium to the patient. *At this time one must do nothing but wait until there is a feeling of peace and harmony. A neutral point will be reached, followed by a long three to four minute pause; and then another neutral point followed by another three to four minute long pause.* The patient 'sinks' more and more, step by step. And, eventually, one will reach the still point, a moment when nothing other than the PRM is perceived – not only in the patient, but in the whole room. (Jealous, 2000, Patients Neutral No. 1, track 14)

The patient will need fewer treatments and the time between each will be longer as this way of working is more enduring and has a more profound effect.

A fervent admirer of Dr Sutherland, Dr Jealous studied the compression of the 4th ventricle in depth and over many years developed a new technique that he called the expansion of the 4th ventricle (EV4). This involves a very simple, formidably effective technique. 'We do not direct the tide,' said Jealous, 'we synchronize it with the movement that is already there, regardless of how small it is.'

He explains this technique on one of his CDs:

What you will get is a very prolonged inhalation phase [of the 4th ventricle] that could go on for 10 to 15 minutes. […] It will go to a point where it will kind of build up a little bit more inhalation, a little bit more and then all of a sudden in a lot of cases it will go 'ssssssss,' and the patient will take in a deep breath involuntarily that is completely synchronized with a similar deep breath in primary respiration. All of a sudden the boundaries of the inhalation phase dissolve. And after that, things get very very quiet; usually there is a still point. The body comes to a point of balance and it rests for a while in neutral. It's not breathing in, it's not breathing out. It's just there, balanced upon the stillness from which it emerged at conception. And after a while we start to get inhalation and exhalation of the primary respiration. Now if you are successful with that EV4, it's going to take a number of days for that treatment to really sink it. You've just turned the therapeutic process on, so to re-evaluate the patient now in terms of tissue motion makes no intelligent sense. The treatment just began, so you let the patient go home for X number of days, depending on the depth of the therapeutic process that you perceive, and then have them come back. It's amazing how many symptoms, even in severely neurologically impaired kids, start to mould themselves into constructive function with this first treatment. (Jealous, 2000, EV4 No 1, track 17)

First of all, Jealous says, return your patient to a normal state; then, if required, treat him. Apply techniques, treat the bones, etc. But first of all, return the body to normality.

Jealous used lots of pauses; there is a pause before, during and after his treatment. In every case, rather than direct or disturb the body, one must allow it to act and react. This is authentic self-regulation.

### Andrew Taylor Still DO: 'Find it, fix it, and leave it alone; Nature will do the rest'

According to Paul Chauffour DO, Still used the following five methods of treatment:

–Simple techniques. Still used the same principles of muscle stretching and articular mobilization to treat all regions of the body.

–Direct techniques. The 'good old doctor' always tried to correct lesions directly, by applying a force that was opposite to the resistance.

–Techniques without 'thrust.' Still worked on various tissue restrictions which locked the osteopathic lesion, without any forced manipulation (thrust).

–Rapid techniques. Corrections were made in a very short adjustment period, at most a few minutes. This limited excessive intervention once the tissue was released. (This would explain 'Find it, fix it, and leave it alone').

–Comfortable techniques. As much out of respect for the patient as in the interest of efficiency, the methods of Still were never dangerous, aggressive, or painful. (Chauffour and Prat, 2002, p. 43)

Steve Paulus DO provides a slightly more detailed explanation of the expression 'Find it, fix it, and leave it alone':

The first of the three phrases is easily understood and does not require any philosophical arguments. 'Find it,' refers to finding a precise cause. This implies a complete understanding of anatomy and consideration for pathophysiological laws of causes and effects as well as the ability to distinguish the normal from the abnormal in the body.

The second part, 'fix it,' relates to the patient who came to us and asked for help because he has not been able to 'fix' the problem himself. This means removing the material or physical cause for whatever distortion or obstruction is preventing the organism's normal functions.

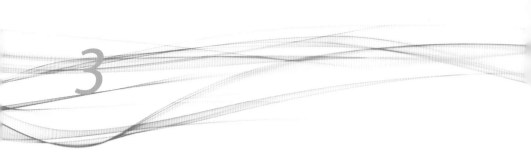

The third part, 'leave it alone,' requires us to have confidence in the role Nature plays in healing the patient. Dr Still used to say: 'Fix it' is not a cure in itself; Healing is brought about when you 'leave it alone'. You, osteopath technicians, can only adjust the abnormal condition. Nature will do the rest.' It is not the osteopath who heals the patient. (Paulus, 2009)

Still did not offer physiological explanations per se, nor the precise length of time the patient should be allowed to rest, but he knew that he must wait and allow the self-regulating process (the miracle of Nature) to occur.

Paulus adds:

It is neither the osteopath's determination nor his ego that heals; it is the internal process of self-regulation.[3]

Those who work this way (find it, fix it, leave it) are the least arrogant therapists. *They are required to deliberately wait, regardless of which type of self-regulation is sought.* [...] Those who do not do this are not real osteopaths, they are technicians of bio-mechanics.

These points add weight to the hypothesis of the necessity of the pause.

More about this quote 'Find it, fix it, and leave it alone; Nature will do the rest ': It is important to know that it is not from the writings of Still. As Jane Eliza Stark DOMP, mentioned, several quotes attributed to Still are taken from the memoirs of H.H. Gravett published in 1948 (Stark, 2012). Gravett speaks about, among other things, A.T. Still's conference at the American School of Osteopathy in 1896. At this conference, Still apparently said: 'It is important that you find it, and it is just as important to know when you have fixed it and to leave it alone, nature will do the rest' (Gravett, 1948).

In 1925, 23 years before H.H. Gravett's publication, this famous quote attributed to Still is found on page 25 of a book entitled *Doctor A.T. Still, Founder of Osteopathy* written by Michael A. Lane (1925).

Other traces of this quotation, dated 1910, can be found on a postcard on which Dr. A.T. Still appears (Fig. 3.6 A and B).

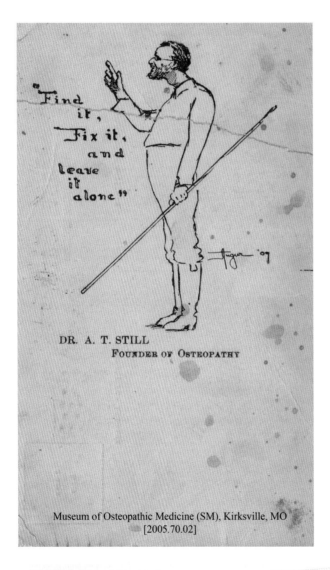

"Find it, Fix it, and leave it alone"

DR. A. T. STILL
FOUNDER OF OSTEOPATHY

Museum of Osteopathic Medicine (SM), Kirksville, MO
[2005.70.02]

**FIGURE 3.6 A**

Postcard with a drawing of Andrew Taylor Still, with a stamp from Kirksville dated 2010. Reproduced with the permission of the Museum of Osteopathic Medicine[sm], Kirksville, MO

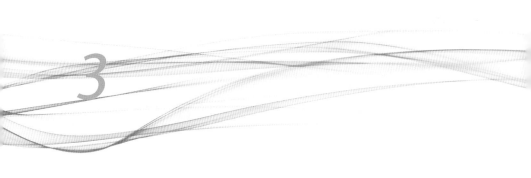

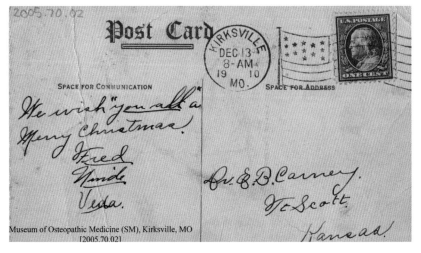

Museum of Osteopathic Medicine (SM), Kirksville, MO
[2005.70.02]

**FIGURE 3.6 B**

## Finding common ground

Each of these authors, each of these osteopaths, published, said and recorded a huge amount of information from which we have here selected a few lines. But it is possible to realize that, although expressed in different words, all seem to evoke the same principle: slow down, wait or even stop.

To go back to Still's famous quote and apply it to the context of this book, we could say that:

*–Find it* implies that the osteopath must not only find the cause of the problem in the patient's body in compliance with the rules of anatomy and physiology, but he must also assess the patient's social, economic, and emotional situation, assess his lifestyle and find elements which increase his allostatic load.

*–Fix it* requires that, in addition to removing the material or physical cause through osteopathic treatment (or other), the patient must also

be educated, made aware of the social and emotional situation, and things in his lifestyle which can tax the body to such a point where, alone, treatment is more palliative than curative. Allostatic load is reduced through both treatment and education.

–*Leave it alone* seems to imply precisely the moment of pause, in which no other intervention is carried out and where the body must activate its self-regulation process?

–*Nature will do the rest* would be equivalent to the quote attributed to Hippocrates 'vis medicatrix naturae,' which means that left alone, the body can often heal by itself. This quote was used by Walter B. Cannon when he developed the concept of homeostasis.

**Find the physical, physiological, emotional and contextual cause.**

**Treat the cause, and reduce the harmful effects of the environment on the physiology.**

**Allow time for the body to find its path to normalization.**

**Thus, balance can be restored.**

**Try it!**

### Notes

[1.] Sutherland seems to have shared this opinion. Tricot (2005, p. 162) cites Sutherland when addressing the compression of the 4th ventricle which, by slowing down exchanges and diffusing the CSF toward the periphery, acts as a penetrating oil: 'I want to draw your attention to the benefits of the cerebrospinal fluid in the treatment of chronic lesions in the spinal cord. I call it "penetrating oil," like the oil used for old rusted joints. A mechanic does not try to turn rusted old nuts and bolts with a key. He begins by applying a drop or two of oil into the threads. Once the oil has acted, the mechanic can turn the nut and bolt with his fingers without damaging the threads. By redirecting the tide toward a very short rhythmic period and this significant exchange of all the fluids in the body, you can progressively lubricate chronic situations and return them to normal, functional conditions. The fibrosis will also diminish and normal muscle tissue will in time reappear.'

[2.] Body physiology according to Rollin Becker: total capacity of an individual to create health and to resist or adapt to trauma and/or disease (Becker, 2001, p. 80).

[3.] The website, www.interlinea.com, from which this reference was taken in 2009, is no longer online. It is therefore impossible to validate the notes. I therefore wrote to Steve Paulus in order to obtain an exact reference for the text in question and he kindly answered that as this quote is one of the fundamentals of osteopathy, each of us must find its significance.

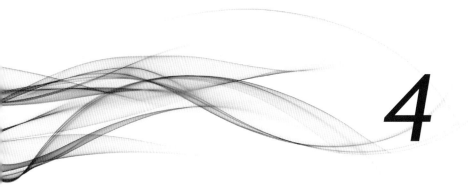

# Integration time in other manual therapies

There are manual therapies which mark, in an obvious manner, one or more stopping periods during treatment. We can name the Strain–Counterstrain method, the Bowen method and chiropractic techniques which, in B.J. Palmer's time of 1936, insisted on the importance of giving the body an integration period.

Having sent an email to several of my French therapist colleagues asking if they knew of other therapies in which a pause was integrated, I received dozens of replies. Among these replies, mention is made of various therapeutic methods, manual or otherwise, which speak of a 'pause' sometimes during the session, but more often afterwards. Obviously, there is acupuncture, but also NST (neurostructural integration technique), myotherapy, microkinesitherapy, connective tissue massage, neural massage, energy physiotherapy, the Furter method, chromatotherapy, sophrology, EMDR (eye movement desensitization and reprocessing), the Niromathe method, the Moneyron method, the Feldenkrais method, the Danis Bois method, trigger point therapy and yoga. Some therapists who practice these methods talk about and apply pauses intuitively, as if it were normal to stop for a while or to slow down.

We feel it and we do it.

## Chiropractic

B.J. Palmer, son of D.D. Palmer the founding father of chiropractic, was an advocate of the post-treatment pause. He did not have any precise scientific explanation for this, however, in his experience, he found he could not do without it. He had 'resting rooms' where patients lay still for *'no less than an hour'* after an adjustment. The patients had to rest in a small, calm, peaceful room and sleep if possible. According to Palmer, omitting this part of the treatment would render the adjustment temporary, and any possibility of a permanent outcome would be lost.

It takes a second for the concussion of forces to deliver the movement or motion which will produce or reduce a vertebral subluxation. It would be folly, following adjustment, for case to arise from adjusting table, begin twisting, jerking, wrenching, and straining the new-normal position of corrected vertebrae; to put muscles, cartilages, ligaments 'to a test to see if it will stay put'. Case must rest 'not less than one hour'; relax, sleep if possible, in quiet, peaceful rest room provided for that purpose.

By failing to lie down, the adjustment has temporary value decreasing its health restorative value. The rest room increases the constant of correction and decreases liability of traumatic variable slipping back to old abnormal position (Palmer, 1936, p. 174).

The resting rooms should have comfortable beds, soft pillows, clean sheets for each patient, soft light, upholstered doors, carpets in the hallways, tiles in each room and doors with locks. The rooms should be kept warm in winter and cool in summer.

## Strain-Counterstrain

This treatment for somatic dysfunctions was developed by Lawrence Jones DO FAAO. He defined Strain-Counterstrain as 'a passive positional procedure that places the body in a position of maximum comfort, thereby relieving pain by reducing and arresting inappropriate proprioceptor activity which maintains somatic dysfunction' (Jones, 1995).

This definition of Strain–Counterstrain applies to aberrant neuromuscular reflexes in the tissue. More specifically, the primary proprioceptor nerve endings are identified as transmitting false information to the central nervous system, maintaining somatic dysfunction. The therapist affects the central nervous system by passively positioning the patient's dysfunctioning limb in a way which limits pain, tension or restrictive barriers as much as possible. This results in the maximum shortening of the implicated muscle and its proprioceptors and therefore a progressive reduction in the neuromuscular discharge.

Thus Lawrence Jones's hypothesis is that an aberrant afferent flux originating in the muscle spindle produces a reflex spasm in the muscle that sets the joint in a certain direction and resists any other attempt to reset it in a neutral position.

During his experiments, Jones observed that a very slow return to a neutral position was key to the resulting positional release. If the

# Integration time in other manual therapies

patient were moved too quickly, particularly in the first 15 degrees of movement, the benefits of the positioning would be lost. Also, after originally having supported the patient in a position of release for 20 minutes, he was systematically able to reduce this period to 90 seconds. Any period less than 90 seconds produced incoherent results. But any period over 90 seconds did not seem to increase the benefits for the patient.

However, maintaining the position for 90 seconds allowed the neuromuscular spindles to slow down the frequency of the afferent discharges. A slow, deliberate return to a neutral position prevented re-excitation of the previously spasmed muscle. 'The shortened spindle nevertheless continues to fire, despite the slackening of the main muscle, and the CNS is gradually able to turn down the gamma discharge, and, in turn, enables the muscle to return to 'easy neutral' at its resting length' (Korr, 1947).

## Dr Snow's mechanical vibration and Dr Gregory's spondylotherapy

The website 'Early American Manual Therapy' is a mine of information about the development of manual therapies at the beginning of the last century, in the United States in particular. Unabridged versions of many important books, such as the works of Littlejohn, Still, Palmer and Louisa Burns can be found there. Some of these books were written by people less well known to osteopaths, such as Dr Snow and Dr Gregory. These two medical doctors both described methods which use vibrations and require a pause and an integration time.

### Dr Snow's mechanical vibration, 1912

In Dr Snow's time, the public and professionals had already turned their attention toward natural treatment methods as a means of avoiding medication. As a consequence, progress in manual therapies was made every year. One of these forms of therapy, the mechanical vibration method, got a lot of attention.

'Mechanical vibration or vibrating massage,' as defined by doctors at the time, was any type of vibration, whether it be a back and forth movement on one plane or from top to bottom, percussion, oscillation,

**4**

a reoccurring or gyrating vibration. According to the theory, when a vibration is induced on a group of particles of matter, a succession of waves forms. The distance between two succeeding wave crests is called the wavelength. When many waves transmit their pulse signal to a given spot, their impact produces interference. This interference can increase, diminish or inhibit movement. The speed of wave transmission increases according to the elasticity of the medium. Thus, each tissue or organ can only receive the waves that their elasticity permits.

The pause during the treatment had to be as long as or twice as long as the treatment of a specific part of the body. When the technique of interrupted vibrations was used, the intermission periods had to be as long as or twice as long as the periods of contact. A rest period of at least 30 minutes was needed at the end of the session for the 'setting and perpetuity' of the benefits of the vibrations.

It was suggested that this method should not be used less than 30 minutes after a meal and that, if the mechanical vibrations were to be applied to the abdomen, it would be better to wait an hour.

According to Dr Snow, the general physiological effects of the mechanical vibrations were numerous. 'They had an effect on biomechanics, thermo-regulation, the metabolism and reflexes. The most noticeable effects were the biochemical changes that occurred after treatments' (Snow, 1912). This stimulation seemed to have an effect on chronic diseases when the most common medicines of the time had had little impact. After treatment, profound biochemical changes occurred that could only have been brought about by the vibrations.

The treatment would only be effective if the following criteria were respected:

1. The vibration had to be sufficiently long and rapid. The pressure exerted could not be painful, so the patient's pain tolerance had to be respected.

2. The rapidity and the pressure were determined by the patient's resistance.

3. The interruptions used with the interrupted vibration method had to be limited so as not to exhaust the nerve.

4.  The rest intervals had to be as long as or twice as long as the duration of the contact in order to ensure the perpetuity and the permanence of the effects.

### Spondylotherapy, Alva Emery Gregory MD 1922

Although there were only 10 years between the work of Gregory and Snow, the Great War had changed everything. Technological and scientific discoveries came thick and fast: 'The man with a subconscious mind needs waking up, as it requires a fully conscious mind to keep pace with the progress being made in the healing art, as it is advancing today at rapid speed' (Gregory, 1922).

Normally, says Gregory, there is perfect equilibrium in the amount and efficiency of the nerve impulses and the consequent vital energy generated by and originating within the various nerve centers contained in the brain and spinal cord.

In normal conditions, there is no interference with the generation of vital energy in the nerve centers or with the transmission of vital impulses by motor nerves from the brain and spinal centers where they originate, outward to the various viscera or parts which these transmitting nerves ramify and supply.

Normal conditions are the fundamental requirement for perfect health and efficient auto-protection (the word homeostasis was not well known at this time) which will maintain health as long as these ideal physiological conditions continue. Variations which occur, as well as perturbations at nerve level, lead to an imbalance in function, resulting in disease.

'In sickness,' he said, 'the balance of the nervous system and the nerves is always disturbed.' He therefore uses a technique of percussion which he calls spondylotherapy, which consists of stimulating the spine at specific areas, using staccato pulses (SP) or a current of sine waves (CSW).

The application of the method is described in the texts that Dr Gregory left behind (Gregory, 1922).

# 4

Below are his findings:

–As a general rule, CSW or SP methods carried out rapidly or brief application of pressure on nerves, are more stimulating than continuous and excessive applications, and will have a greater impact on the constriction and the contraction of the viscera.

–CSW and SP methods carried out slowly have a sedative effect and are as effective, if not more so, than when they are carried out rapidly especially if the aim is to inhibit a function or activate a gland.

–*The most effective stimulation is achieved using 10 to 20 rapid impulses per second over 30 seconds, followed by a 30-second pause. This is then repeated again for 30 seconds with a 30-second rest period and so on for a total of five to 10 minutes.*

## The Bowen technique

Thomas Ambrose (Tom) Bowen developed this manual technique in the 1950s. According to him, the ideal therapeutic technique was one which would stimulate the system to rebalance the malfunctions resulting from tissue disruption (Tremblay, 2007). We believe that his way of working, going from one patient to another, meant that pauses lasting a few minutes came about in his treatments. This 'accidental' pause turned out to be very beneficial for his patients, who experienced rapid improvements after only a few sessions.

This therapy thus integrates moments of silence during which the organism undergoes a feedback process allowing it to react to the given stimulation. Only one given impulse is perceived by the central nervous system; it reacts only to this impulse for a certain period of time. The therapist applying the Bowen method does not keep his hands on the patient; he does not therefore 'feel' the moment when the nervous system has completed its adjustment (see the sections in Chapter 3 on Dr Becker and Dr Jealous). He does however ask his patient to inform him when he no longer feels anything in particular in his body. This 'silence' in the body could perhaps be compared to Becker's 'moment of calm' or Jealous's 'quiet point', both different from the still points and often preceding them.

# Integration time in other manual therapies

As long as the patient perceives the slightest sensation, regardless of the type of sensation or where it is felt in the body (which means as long as the insular cortical area is stimulated), the therapist does not touch the patient. This allows him to isolate the stimulation without interrupting the neurological process under way.

With his hands, the therapist sends information to the CNS through the skin receptors and receptors in muscles and tendons. Since each receptor requires a specific type of stimulation, the Bowen gesture must be very precise and focused. While information is being transmitted to the CNS, the Bowen therapist does not decide on the outcome. It seems to be the CNS, in accordance with the patient's priority physiological needs, which is the driving force, triggering the processes which will lead the body to self-regulate. It also appears that the pause is the key element which allows the CNS to initiate the normalization process. This is not specific to the Bowen technique as all manual therapies use the same afferents toward the CNS nerve receptors and subsequent physiology is the same for all patients, regardless of the technique used. But what is unique in the Bowen method is the emphasis placed on this somato-insulo-sensory integration time, which must last at least two minutes, and occurs several times during each session.

## Microkinesitherapy

According to Daniel Grosjean, founder of microkinesitherapy,

> One of the goals of microkinesitherapy is to solicit the repair mechanisms in the body which act when the body stops its activity and rests, probably resulting in the idea of a 'pause'. We find this 'pause' in the therapeutic gesture which consists of reproducing the attack experienced by a muscular or mesoblastic structure (ligament, tendon, capsule) during a traumatic aetiology which stretched these structures beyond their natural elasticity and, therefore, has not regained its physiological functions after this forced stretching. (Grosjean, 2014)

'The therapist reproduces this stretching in the structure until he feels that he can go no further, feeling the resistance of the tissue beyond the amplitude reached; then doing nothing but maintaining this stretch, he waits for the response from the organism. This appears after a pause of varying length, which we can set to about one second per year, largely depending on how old the lesion is.

'During this period, the therapist does nothing; he leaves the organism to set off its repair mechanism. In microkinesitherapy, we say that this period is where the therapist 'does nothing' therefore allowing the organism to 'do something'.

'But we see that the recuperative pause does not occur during the session, but after it, during the night following it. This is the best biological time for repair; the period of deep sleep during which the body repairs and puts order into its structures and functions' (Grosjean, 1984).

## Dermoneuromodulation (DNM)

In an article by Diane Jacobs we read: "The word 'dermoneuromodulation' simply means skin/nervous system/change." It does not imply that the practitioner is the one 'doing' something called 'change' 'to' something anatomical in another person. It does not exclude the nervous system of the patient as change agent under its own auspices, thus DNM is as close to being an interactive model of manual care, as opposed to an operator model, as any kind of manual therapy approach can be, while still handling the bodies of other (live, conscious) people. Other than 'skin', the surface all of us touch regardless of whatever else we might conjecture about what we are doing/affecting/handling, sensory endings, and cutaneous nerves; there is no mention of 'tissue'." (Jacobs, 2012).

So, first, we all work on skin and its receptors. And we inform, we do not 'adjust.'

Without explaining the physiology of the waiting time in her approach, Diane Jacobs insists on taking her time while treating, and making pauses at specific moments. For example, in the description of the technique, she says:

Wait. After about 20 seconds, check with the patient to see if the spot feels more comfortable to them, by poking it a bit and asking them to give you sensory feedback. Usually, it is better, but wait in that position for another minute or two. Remember this pain, like all pain and brain function, especially hindbrain functional change, is a process through time, like all of nature, not a machine with an on-off switch. It takes time for a new pattern to establish itself. **Time is what your patient needs from you**. It is humbling, but the truth is that's all they really need from you, once you've got their layers lined back up with themselves comfortably. (Jacobs, 2009)

## The Niromathe method

Niromathe is a vibratory method developed by Dr Raymond Branly, osteopath, and Thierry Vandorme DO.

As far as Dr Branly is concerned, osteopathic techniques are in fact on neither bone nor muscle nor ligament nor tendon nor fascia nor skin. Whatever they are, they in fact address Tenso-Modulator Elements (TME) located between the skin and the deeper structures.

These TMEs deprogram by 'sticking' to the skin. Their detachment leads, at the same time, to their reprogramming and the instantaneous disappearance of the osteopathic lesion.

It is as if the blockage, the 'seizing' of the joint, were not located at the joint itself, or even in the muscles, but were the result of a 'cutaneous attachment' at the TME: the articulation cannot turn right because the skin cannot be stretched to the right.

In its application, Niromathe slows down the gesture when it reaches maximum amplitude and applies a pause of a few seconds after each move. This brief stop allows time for the wavelength, induced by the vibration, to achieve its goal without interference from other vibrations (Branly, n.d.).

## We make pauses because we feel we should

Virtually all manual therapies speak of stops or slowing down periods, without trying to explain them; as if it were natural to sometimes slow down or stop. Even in nature, there are those stopping times. Times

# 4

when we significantly reduce the amount of external stimuli to let the body integrate and react to those it received in previous moments. Sleep is a good example. Among other things, it allows the body to regenerate and recover its homeostatic balance. We know when we have to sleep, and we do so, even if we are not aware of the physiological details of the homeostatic regulation and other normalizations which occur.

But this is a long pause, after exposure to stimuli over several hours. Let's take another example, where the exposure time is shorter, such as visiting the Louvre Museum. Unless one is gifted with an extraordinary capacity for integration, it is practically impossible to visit, even in part, passing in front of each of the works one after the other while remaining totally focused, without stopping. We cannot at the same time see, understand and integrate all of Picasso's works if each is held one by one before our eyes without any pause. We will have seen them, but we will not have understood or integrated them. The amount of information is too vast; we feel we need to stop.

The information that the patient receives during an osteopathy or manual therapy session follows on and accumulates. What can we do to ensure that all the information is perceived, discriminated and integrated by the CNS? How can the CNS understand what the therapist is trying to tell him using somesthesic language if the therapist is not aware of what the CNS needs in order to understand?

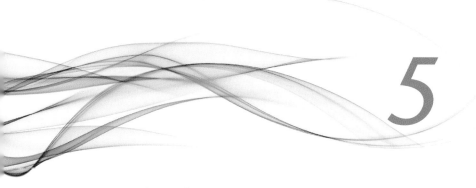

# Conceptual analysis

## Different types of pause

Through presentation of these various manual methods of care, it seems increasingly clear that there is not just one type of pause, but at least three, each with specific features and serving very different purposes: the homeostasis anticipation pause, the 'still point' and the somato-insulo-sensory integration time.

### *The homeostasis anticipation pause*

We could also call this an accompanying pause toward homeostasis. This 'pause' is well known to osteopaths. It involves maintaining a fulcrum in order that the organism can inform itself of the change, self-assess and trigger a rebalancing around this new state.

Let us again quote Rollin Becker's experience taken from Jacques Andreva Duval's book:

> The practitioner chooses the area which he is going to treat first. To determine the 'key point', he uses the symptoms described by the patient or any other test which may indicate an area requiring special attention.

> The practitioner places his hand(s) on or under the patient's body on the tissue at the key point and applies a moderate degree of controlled compression in the direction of the involved tissue. He has thus established a fulcrum in contact with the physiology of the patient's body [...].

> The physiology of the patient's body begins to exhibit balanced rhythmic exchanges in the chosen tissue. This activity is perceived by the practitioner's sense of touch.

> The practitioner's point of contact does not remain rigidly and passively attached to the patient's body: it is certainly a silent contact, but it is also alert, alive, receptive. The hands remain supple; they adapt slowly to changes in movements of balance and rhythmic

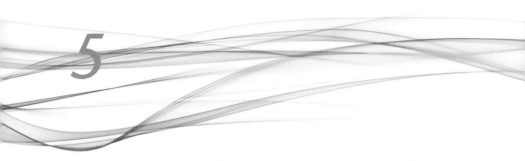

exchanges; they mould to the changes that occur in the body of the patient [...].

> Through his point of contact, the practitioner supports the tissue to its point of equilibrium until it produces a modification and relaxation of rhythmic exchange activity. He maintains that contact until the rhythmic and balanced activity of involved tissue has indicated to him that the elements of the key point are relaxed and working in a healthier way to the heart of the patient's physiology. (Duval, 2008, p. 67)

This moment before the high point, which is maintained by a fulcrum and that leads to homeostasis, is particular to osteopathy.

Continuing with the comparison to music, we could call this moment 'the physiological anacrusis.' In music, an anacrusis is the note or sequence of notes which precede the first downbeat in a bar. It is also a form of writing in music and poetry which indicates that the work begins with a silence or a breath.

### The pause as a 'still point'

There are various types of 'still point'.

### The physiological still point and the resolution still point

As we have seen already, Pierre Tricot, in his book *Approche tissulaire de l'ostéopathie*, describes two still points: the physiological still point and the resolution still point (Tricot, 2005, p. 117).

The physiological still point is the one which is inherent in normal physiology and which occurs when any alternating phenomenon occurs. It is also a moment when the energy potentiates before movement begins again, for example, slack tide. The resolution still point is the moment when the structure, having finished releasing the retained energy, is waiting before starting to move again. It is essential, said Pierre Tricot, that the practitioner respects this and waits, and this wait can last a while.

### The induced still point

John E. Upledger describes a still point variant:

> It is a question of determining the direction of greatest ease and range of physiological craniosacral motion. Follow this motion to its physiological end point, and resist its return. Take up the slack with each ensuing cycle until a still point of craniosacral system function is reached. After the still point is ended and improved craniosacral system activity is resumed, the therapist monitors and evaluates the new physiological motion patterns. The still point may last a few seconds to a few minutes. When it is over, the craniosacral system will resume its motion, usually with a better symmetry and a larger amplitude. (Upledger and Vredevoogd, 2014 [1983], p. 41)

The difference between the still point described by John E. Upledger and the one described by Pierre Tricot or Rollin Becker lies in the fact that during the application of the Upledger technique, the practitioner resists return of mobility until a still point is obtained while Becker and Tricot talk about accompaniment by a fulcrum to reach the still point. Both techniques, however, lead to a similar goal, reaching a moment of tranquillity where the patient's physiology is able to restore its homeostatic balance.

### The spontaneous still point

According to Rollin Becker, still points can occur in other parts of the body, places which the therapist does not touch. 'You're quietly working on, listening to, some area in a patient, and all of a sudden, you're aware of something happening elsewhere. Well, it had to have gone through a still point for that to have happened. But you weren't in the area at the time it took place. You can be aware of the fact that the change took place, that something went through a still point, but you weren't the author of it' (Becker, 2006, p. 69).

### *One way of recognizing a still point*

James Jealous:

> The body comes to a point of balance and it rests for a while in neutral. It's not breathing in, it's not breathing out. It's just there,

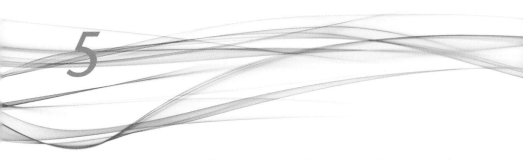

5

balanced upon the stillness from which it emerged at conception. (Jealous, 2000, EV4 No 1, track 17)

This reminds us a lot of what happens during deep meditation, where time and space no longer count. It also elicits the moment before falling asleep or waking up, where all is calm, where one feels completely well, completely composed, heavy and light at the same time. These seem to be the moments when communication goes beyond words, where the depth of sensations opens to a happy place, of total well-being.[1]

During an osteopathy session, therefore, the body can reach a point where it must stop and where further stimulation could disturb this moment of calm which is required for self-normalization to occur.

The description of the occurrence of a still point according to James Jealous may also seem familiar to other manual therapists who do not practice osteopathy. Indeed, it is very common to see this phenomenon in patients when the therapist has been careful to take a pause during the application of their method. Rollin Becker also said that a still point can occur in an area where the therapist has not touched: 'A still point is a physiologic balancing act that the body physiology of any patient is going through. It can occur anytime, anywhere, anyhow. It probably occurs spontaneously in patients during a good night's sleep or something like that' (Becker, 2006, p. 69). The following two questions are troubling, but must be asked:

–Do we always need to keep our hands on the patient in order for the still point to occur?

–Does a somato-insulo-sensory integration time have something to do with the occurrence of a still point?

It is interesting to read in more detail in Appendix V what the therapist can feel and observe during a still point.

### Somato-insulo-sensory integration time

In music, the metacrusis happens after crusis, after the downbeat. It is the silence; the one which allows you to hear. This silence occurs during the symphony, intensifying the impact, and also at the end of the symphony, as a reminder which can last for several hours or several days, making the impact felt during the experience of listening to the music persist.

In our case we interpret this as a moment of silence when no further stimulation is added, a time when the body disposes of, integrates and responds to the latest information it has received.

Almost all manual therapies require the patient to remain tranquil for a few days after the session, thus allowing full integration of the effects.

Some therapies rely on this pause during the session. We saw Lawrence Jones's 'Strain-Counterstrain' method where it is suggested that the muscle be maintained in its shortest position for as long as it takes for neuromuscular spindle activity to stop, so at least 90 seconds, before gradually laying the limb down, whilst avoiding reactivation of the neuromuscular spindles. The muscle then returns to its original length in its rest position.

There is also the Niromathe method which uses the principle of tissue vibration, as does Dr Snow's method that we saw earlier. Niromathe slows down the move when its amplitude is at a maximum and pauses for a few seconds after each of these moves, giving time for the vibration-induced wavelength to reach its goal without interference from other vibrations.

For Diane Jacobs (dermoneuromodulation), we all work on skin and its receptors. She insists on the fact that, as therapists, we inform, we do not 'adjust'. Pain is a process through time, like all of nature, not a machine with an on–off switch. It takes time for a new pattern to establish itself. Time is what our patient really needs from us.

There is another therapy where pauses are key to its efficiency: it is the Bowen method. Although Tom Bowen did not explain this pause, certain people focused on the need for pauses. Indeed, empirically and without further studies to support these findings, but given the feedback from hundreds of therapists over thousands of treatments, it has been found that the less the therapist makes pauses, and the shorter these pauses are, the less the session brings about the desired results. Conversely, the more the therapist stops to let the body react as the session continues, the more this pause time is respected, the better the results and the stronger the patient's responses. Since the therapist does not have hands on the subject during this therapeutic pause and therefore cannot feel the moment of resolution, it was important to find a way to 'measure' how long this break should last. Tom Bowen proposed two minutes, intuitively we think; this does respect, however, the physiology of the neuromuscular spindle which takes at least 90 seconds to cease its activity. It was suggested that this pause continue for as long as the subject felt something 'happening' inside his body, a sign of activity in the insular cortex (Craig, 2009).

In all three cases, Bowen, Niromathe or Jones, these are somato-insulo-sensory integration moments, interspaced between the various manipulations or techniques used: the time when the therapist waits, does not activate, does not move, he lets the body react.

## The appropriateness of a pause in osteopathy in relation to physiology

Rollin Becker himself emphasized the importance of respecting the time the physiology of the CNS takes to respond to a specific stimulation:

> In the fulcrum point approach, you lay your hands under a patient to examine an area of osteopathic strain and establish your fulcrum point; you get your hand against that tissue so you have a hand lever hold on the area you are examining. The patient's body mechanism initiates a response — the simple reflex arc, which is relatively quick — into the core and out again. But it also initiates the responses of the central and autonomic nervous systems that go to the brain, participate in all the sensory interchange in the brain, and produce an outflow that finds its way back down through all these tissues. *This occurs more slowly, taking a matter of seconds or minutes.*

> With your hand under this patient, you feel this gentle give and take, the swinging of these tissues. You are observing the responses of the central and autonomic nervous systems to this fulcrum point

that you have established on this patient, and this tissue movement is coming from the body's anatomy and physiology. It is not the patient that is doing the moving. What initiates the total thing into motion is the patient's nervous system sending the orders down to all the components within this tissue mechanism, which is the environmental energy and osteopathic lesion. The fulcrum point of the operator has initiated this mechanism into acting.

When you establish a fulcrum point and then apply a little pressure to it, you have applied strength, and it is the responses of the patient's segmental, central, and autonomic nervous systems that you are picking up as the tissue begins its pattern of action. When the mechanism starts, it tends to wind its way in toward the point of balance which is correct for that anatomical-physiological-pathological configuration. The mechanism comes to a still point, makes a change, and begins to unwind. (Becker, 2001, p. 117)

Rollin Becker says that the CNS plays a key role in the normalization initiated by the osteopath's hands. *The body will carry out its normalization if given the opportunity to do so.*

The neuroendocrine system is very complex: science has yet to uncover all of its secrets. However, it seems that many clues point to the physiological significance of pausing after the body has received information from treatment therapies which use somatosensory pathways. Below some key points from Chapter 1 will be used in an attempt to formulate principles which could become scientific research hypotheses using the deductive method.

*1. The nervous system and the endocrine system are bi-directional methods of communication.*

This could therefore be called a dialogue, a means of communicating rather than imposing a point of view. In philosophy, to dialogue is to discuss together. This is useful for the osteopath who seeks to stimulate the self-regulatory process. Dialogue assumes that we know and speak the language of the interlocutor and that we allow him to express himself, giving him the time he needs to do so.

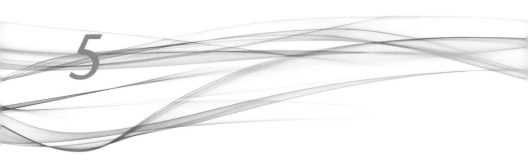

*2. There are three types of exit in the CNS: the motor system, and through the ANS, the smooth muscles or the glands.*

We do not know and cannot control what our interlocutor's response will be. Will it be motor or hormonal in nature? We cannot determine this. We know that somesthesic stimulation can provoke a hormonal response, as we saw with the example of childbirth. We know that nature has provided us with a pause mechanism between contractions. Why? Perhaps to allow time for the receptors in the cervix to recover the action potential, perhaps to allow time for the reticular formation to transmit somesthesic information to the hypothalamus, perhaps to allow time for the reverberating circuits in the hypothalamus to create and release the right amount of oxytocin for the next contraction; perhaps for all of these things. But the example is there and speaks volumes.

*3. The nervous and endocrine systems react to stimuli at different rates. In general, nerve impulses have an effect in a few milliseconds. Responses of the endocrine system are often slower than responses of the nervous system; although some hormones act within seconds, most take several minutes or more (hours) to generate a response. The effects of nervous system activation are generally briefer than those of the endocrine system.*

Reactions can take anywhere from a few milliseconds for a nerve impulse (depending on how it is treated by the reticular formation) to a few seconds, to many hours. Research and the experiences of practicing osteopaths have shown that somesthesic information can provoke hormonal reactions. There are few studies to back this up, which would make it a fascinating research topic. We know that hormonal responses take longer to complete than nerve responses. To optimize results, would it not be advisable to wait two or three minutes after each technique to allow the hypothalamus time to process the possible effects of this stimulation?

A return to homeostatic equilibrium and the maintenance of this equilibrium is a precondition for health. Since we also know that the nerve control centre for biological rhythms is located in the hypothalamus and that it sometimes takes seconds or minutes for the hypothalamus to react, why not give it time?

*4. Even if the physiological threshold of excitation is reached, as long as the perceptive threshold is not reached, the stimulation will not be perceived. Discrimination of stimuli occurs at the reticular formation.*

The role of the cells in the reticular formation is to evaluate the intensity of the nerve messages that converge there, whatever their origin.

The ascending reticular activating system seems to serve as a filter for this influx of sensory information. It attenuates repetitive, familiar or weak signals but allows unexpected, important or intense signals to reach the conscience.

*5. The ascending reticular activating system and the cerebral cortex no doubt neglect 99 % of the sensory stimuli registered by our receptors.*

The more the stimulation is unique, the less interference there is, the more likely it is to be regarded and therefore to pass the barrier of the reticular formation to be conveyed to higher centres.

*6. The reverberating circuit discharges repeatedly for a long moment. At the exit, the signal can last many milliseconds or even minutes. This type of circuit is used by the reticular formation and the autonomous nervous system (which is regulated by the hypothalamus).*

We also know that the reticular formation limits the access of sensory messages from other origins to the cortex by inhibiting corresponding sensory pathways. We can assume that any information, regardless of its origin, which is stronger or more unusual than the information which had initiated the reverberating process, could lead the reticular formation to inhibit the reverberating signal and prioritize the other information. This is why, after applying stimulation, we should allow the time for this message be completely executed before proceeding with further stimulation.

*7. Regardless of which sensory system is activated, there must be a contrast between two stimulations in order for them to be perceived.*

Pausing between stimulations allows for this contrast: black is especially visible on a white background, not so much on a dark blue background.

Sounds are clear if they are not lost amongst other noise. The therapeutic pause could well be the contrast needed for somatosensory inputs.

**8. The most important of the regulatory mechanisms which prevent the brain from information overload is the adapting of receptors. This is where the sensory systems react less to continuous or repeated exposure to a stimulus.**

The pause prevents the receptors from adapting and possibly prevents information overload of the brain.

**9. The thalamus is the principal hub between sensory signals and the cerebral cortex.**

Excitation signals in the thalamus originate in the reticular formation through small, very slow conduction fibers. The excitation effect develops over a few seconds or up to a minute. Only then will the information be transmitted to the cortex. It is astonishing to note that at the heart of the brain, where we would think everything would occur in milliseconds, there are neuronal processes which take some minutes to complete. We have always understood that this was the case for hormone production; however, this was less evident in the case of neuronal processes.

**10. The feelings from the body are each characterized by a distinct sensation which is inherently colored by a strong affect directly associated with a motivation driving behavioral responses needed to maintain the health of the body; in other words, the affective feelings from the body occur concomitantly with motivations for homeostatic behavior.**

From our experience, it may take several seconds, or even minutes, before a sensation is felt in the body after mechanical stimulation. Perhaps we should leave time between mechanical stimuli and allow the body to reach the moment where behavioral responses will develop in order to maintain homeostasis.

To summarize: a reverberating circuit in the brain or in the reticular formation can discharge over several minutes; the transfer of information from the reticular formation to the thalamus and other regions in the brain can take up to a minute; the hypothalamus can take many minutes to synthesize a hormone or a 'releasing factor' following somesthesic stimulation, and homeostatic behavior occurs concomitantly with affective feelings, which may arise several seconds or minutes after mechanical stimuli.

These four reasons would be sufficient cause to seriously reconsider our way of working. But we also know that the more stimulations we make, the less the one we want to emphasize will be perceived as important. The pause makes it possible to isolate the information we deem essential.

*It seems as though the pause... is imposed.*

## The appropriateness of a pause in osteopathy in relation to its philosophy

'... The osteopathic concept can be elevated to a philosophy in the best sense of the term, as it is indeed a study of wisdom taken from the point of view both of knowledge of the human body, and of therapeutic action' (Desjardins, 1993 cited in Saine, 1996, p. 64).

Osteopathy must take into account, amongst other things, the physiology of the body. We have shown that there is a very strong possibility that this moment of pause is important for the integration of information.

What is striking is the use, by many influential osteopaths, (among them some of the 'fathers' of osteopathy – Still, Sutherland, Becker, Jealous, Jones, Tricot, Upledger, Fernandez), of pauses, rest times, time to listen.[2] Each one of these osteopaths has, in his own way, described what he felt and has spoken of 'leaving the patient to rest,' of the 'still point,' a 'moment of calm,' or a 'neutral point.' Even the father of chiropractic, Palmer, had his patients rest for at least an hour after manipulation. If Still did not describe his techniques in his books and did not specify a precise waiting time when he stated, 'Find it, fix it, and leave it alone,' perhaps we should ask ourselves what his students or peers did. It seems that Sutherland made use of 'somato-insulo-sensory pauses,' as did Palmer.

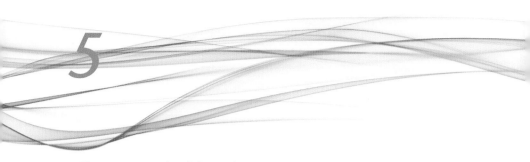

These osteopaths did not describe the neurological processes which could take place during the pause. At that time little was known of neuronal networks, or of hormone production and functions. But today it is possible to show how a pause can affect the organism.

Physiology integrates the pause. Osteopathy also incorporates the pause: we have noticed this through the various techniques studied. Following these observations, and as a result of our research and our experience in the practice of manual therapies which incorporate the therapeutic pause, it seems reasonable to argue that a pause between somesthesic techniques during manual therapy is essential in order for patients' results to be optimized.

## How can the pause be integrated into osteopathic treatments?

The pause can be integrated into osteopathic treatments in the most natural way possible, as all good osteopaths have always done. This is not an additional technique, nor a method that follows a fixed law which must be applied in every case. We have seen how somesthesic stimulation can influence the neuroendocrine system. If we want the osteopathic technique which we have just used on a given patient to have durable effects on the organism, we must leave a pause. Because of this, thanks to this, we leave the time needed for the action to develop completely. We apply the principle of the somato-insulo-sensory integration time, especially when it comes to successive manipulations such as those of hormonal or myofascial chains, or manipulations such as recoil or thrust, etc.

How long should the pause last? Many therapists think that between 90 and 120 seconds are necessary.[3] We agree with this minimum time; however, we add that as long as the patient feels something happening in his body, or as long as the osteopath has not felt normalization in his hands during passive tissue listening, the pause must continue. This method can be applied to all kinds of treatment, and to all patients.

It also seems important to limit other sensory stimuli during manipulation and during pauses, in order to give priority to those of interest. As demonstrated by Pascal Fortier-Poisson in his thesis presented in 2012 at the University of Montreal, 'the overall activity of the subject's somato-sensory cortex is increased if we allow the subject to be attentive to the cutaneous stimulus rather than enduring it whilst performing a visual or auditory task (Fortier-Poisson, 2012). We must therefore take care to reduce or eliminate other stimuli such as noise, strong odors, bright light and temperature variations.

I was made aware of this work during the autumn of 2012, more than three years after writing the thesis which would lead to this book. I suggest the reader take note of the additions to Appendix VI, where the latest research on this subject is cited. I consider this research to be of paramount importance to manual therapy practitioners.

### Notes

[1.] 'O Time, suspend your flight! And you, favored times, Suspend your course! Let us savor the momentary delights. Of the most beautiful of our days!' Lamartine. It is like the moment when the eagle or the albatross is suspended in the air, in complete osmosis between air currents and gravity/weight, time which seems 'never-ending' and where lightness takes on an intense strength, composition or ecstatic combination of time and space (Racano, 2014).

[2.] And it seems that there were others, such as Bénichou for example, as witnessed by some of our students.

[3.] Which also corresponds to the period of time required for a large tide cycle such as was proposed by Rollin Becker.

# 6 CONCLUSION

Osteopathy is an art. Like music, visual arts, literary arts and other artistic expressions without mentioning them all. The winemaker, for example, in the development of his wine, must respect several pause times. The vine's pause during the winter when the winemaker takes the opportunity to prune. The pause of the newly pressed juice, which will be left to ferment in vats; then will be put into barrels to allow yeast and bacteria to work; it takes a long time; then this juice becomes wine which will be bottled where the 'pause', the wait may be even longer in order to develop all the awaited qualities of the wine. The winemaker is an artist. His senses tell him when to harvest, how long to leave it in vats, how much time in barrels, etc. Winemaking is carried out over a period of time, during which the biochemical and physiological processes inherent in its production can occur. And then, winemakers will tell you: avoid shaking it. You will then find the quintessence of all those pauses when you open a vintage Meursault Charmes 2002; you might even find yourself living suspended, for a moment, as in a still point …

A conductor does not draw out all the sounds the orchestra can make at the same time. He senses when to bring in a musician or when to tell him to wait. Silence is as important as sound: the clarity of the sound depends on the perfection of the silence on which it rests. The osteopath, as the conductor of somesthesia, can use to his advantage – and most importantly, to the patient's advantage – the moments of anticipation and resolution that are the physiological anacrusis and metacrusis. Physiological anacrusis is the silence which allows the osteopath to hear; physiological metacrusis is the silence which allows the CNS to hear.

Upon reflection, this idea seems too simple to be true. It is like something which is so glaringly obvious, everyone can understand it, and yet we refuse to believe it. Society asks us to perform, to go faster, take on more and more. What if our body, which was born in a completely different context millions of years ago, requires us to slow down a little; what if it wants to take its time? Why is it so shocking to realize that our body wants to take its time? Have there not been moments of respite, slowdowns, periods of immutability that continued for thousands of years during which the planet does not seem to have evolved? Then, suddenly a period of intense activity during which everything seems to be accelerated, and then it plateaus out.

It seems to me that it is very important for us to take time to reflect on the importance of these moments of pause, an integral and essential part of osteopathy, many other therapies, rhythms, cycles, and, quite naturally, of life.

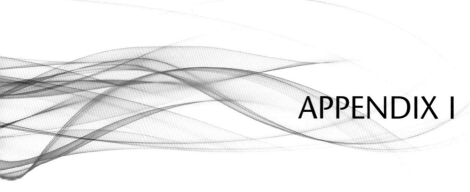

# APPENDIX I

## Synaptic plasticity

Dr Francesco Cerritelli DO, is head of the research department at the *Accademia Italiana Osteopatia Tradizionale* in Pescara, Italy. He also teaches neurophysiology at the same school and is president of the nonprofit making foundation COME Collaboration. After having read my thesis in 2009, he suggested integrating several elements from other research articles: we introduced McEwen and Craig in the chapter on homeostasis. This research allowed me to introduce two new concepts: allostasis and sensual touch. Here are some ideas on synaptic plasticity from Joseph LeDoux's book, which was suggested by Dr Cerritelli.

'The neural basis of learning and memory has been investigated in many different invertebrates (bees, grasshoppers, crayfish, slugs, flies, and various molluscs), but studies of the mollusc Aplysia californica have been particularly thorough and informative. Much of the work on this marine snail has been conducted by Eric Kandel and his students and colleagues at Columbia University and elsewhere. This pioneering research was a major factor in Kandel's receipt of the Nobel Prize in 2000' (LeDoux, 2002).

'Aplysia breathe through gills which are covered by a piece of skin called the mantle. If the mantle is touched lightly, the gill retracts. This defensive reflex protects the gill from injury, and has been the subject of extensive investigation as a behavioral model of learning and memory. The plasticity of other reflexes in Aplysia has also been studied, but the gill-withdrawal reflex will be used to illustrate the basic findings.

'The gill-withdrawal reflex exhibits several forms of learning, including habituation: when non-painful stimuli is applied regularly to the mantle, the amplitude of the gill withdrawal reflex of the animal decreases gradually. Habituation is a form of non-associative learning: a single stimulus is involved, and it is not associated with anything else. Habituation can be reversed rapidly by applying a strong stimulus, such as an electric shock, to some other part of the mollusc's body, such as the tail. After a shock, touching the mantle results in a strong response.

'This exacerbated response is a sensitized response, there has been dis-habituation. The animal then has a kind of learned fear: having

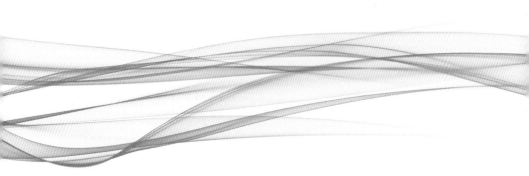

learned to stop worrying about innocuous stimuli, the application of the painful stimulus made it react in an exaggerated manner to other innocuous stimuli. This memory of a painful experience persists if it is renewed: the fear of the painful experience and its associated memory is strengthened by repetition. *One painful experience gives a memory that will last a few minutes, but several painful experiences, spaced in time, give rise to more lasting memories, lasting up to several days'* (Manent, n.d.).

'All forms of gill-reflex learning involve changes in synapses between sensory neurons that receive inputs from the mantle skin and motor neurons that control the gill response. In habituation, for example, the response of the postsynaptic neuron to a presynaptic input weakens, and the gill response diminishes, because the presynaptic terminal comes to release less glutamate. It simply gets depleted. In contrast, in sensitization, the gill reacts more to the same stimulus after the tail is shocked than before because the sensory neuron comes to release more glutamate' (LeDoux, 2002).

How the shock to the snail's tail leads to presynaptic facilitation is explained in detail in Joseph LeDoux's book. What is important for us is to realize that neural pathways are not static, they are changing, enabling learning and participating in the development of long-term memory through somesthesic stimulation.

# APPENDIX II

## Extraocular circadian phototransduction

In 1998, a study was carried out to demonstrate the existence of extraocular circadian phototransduction. 'Biological rhythms are governed by an endogenous circadian clock. The response of the circadian clock in humans to extraocular light exposure was measured using the body temperature and the concentration of melatonin during the circadian cycle before and after the popliteal fossa was exposed to light pulses. A direct link was established between the time of exposure to light and response, and the change in the circadian cycle.' They thus proved 'scientifically' (Campbell and Murphy, 1998), perhaps unintentionally, that somatosensory stimulation (because it is indeed stimulation of receptors in the skin, not the eye, even if it is light) had a direct effect on the endocrine system.

# APPENDIX III

## Dr Guimberteau's observations

Dr Jean-Claude Guimberteau, a plastic surgeon specializing in hand surgery, has studied the fascia. His film, 'Strolling under the skin,' made from videos recorded with an endoscope during surgeries, shows that the collagen network forms a continuous matter composed of billions of tiny disorganized vacuoles apparently arranged in a fractal manner.

'Made of collagen or elastin, these fibrils build microvacuoles filled with gel made of glycosaminoglycan. The collagen fibers which are the armature of each vacuole are linked continuously one to the other and are essentially made up of collagen type 1 (70%) and types 3 and 4, and elastin (20%). There is also a high level of lipids (4%).

'They go off in all directions, without any pre-established plan or any logic. They connect and vibrate against one another. The fibers are only a few microns in diameter. Their length varies widely, giving them a disorganized, chaotic appearance: a series of bundles, a woven grid of stems with gyri (bulges). There are no visible geometric reference points. They criss-cross very distinctly, either in veiled intermediate zones or in veritable fixed knots, solid or mobile anchors that glide with the buoyant force. An extreme close-up reveals lateral modifications on the collagens, suggesting that the chains of proteoglycans are adhesive and linked to the collagens. This is a polyhydric fiber network filled with jelly.'

'The equilibrium of forces in the structure and the capacity to adapt to constraints are the two pillars of dynamic behavior' (Guimberteau, 2005).

Doctor Guimberteau, amongst others, observed that:

–The solicited fibril first responds by withdrawing and then by lengthening, showing a rearrangement of molecules and a capacity to instantaneously recover its original shape. An internal prestressed, spring-like mechanism seems to be solicited first when there is minimal tension.

–Fibers undergoing mechanical solicitation can smoothly divide in space into many fibrils that will disperse and absorb forces more effectively.

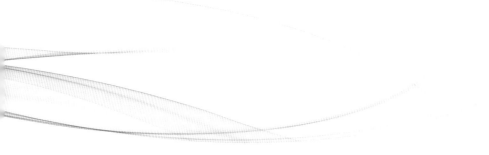

–To respond to the direction of the stress, the biomechanics of the microvacuoles are assisted by the fiber's capacity to migrate around a nodal point, itself encompassing another fiber.

–Fibers, often at their junction with each other, have the ability to either fuse or split in a common gel. This indicates a viscous fluidity capable of friction or attraction which can be explained by covalent bonds.

–Finally, collagens 4 and 6 seem to be able to shear off and reform as if nothing had happened. They also seem to be able to dissociate into several parts, meeting any and every request to move mechanically in space.

Together, says Dr Guimberteau, all the capacities of the fibers combined, supported by the molecular capacity, offer an infinite number of adaptive solutions to any constraint that is imposed. This phenomenon can only be understood in three-dimensional space.

# APPENDIX IV

## The CSF and the collagenic fascial fiber

In the late 1990s, Dr Donald Ingber from the Boston Children's Hospital demonstrated the role of the cell's internal skeleton. Since the 1970s the cytoskeleton was known to be present in the cell. Previously the cell had been pictured as a 'big balloon filled with molasses.' This cytoskeleton was composed of three types of proteins: microfilaments, intermediate filaments and microtubules. However, their role in controlling the shape of the cells was not well-understood. Ingber was able to show the vital role played by microfilaments inside the cell with Buckminster Fuller's tensegrity model. This information, as extraordinary as it was, would have remained incomplete for us osteopaths if he had not brought to light the link between the cytoskeleton and the extracellular matrix: the integrins. These molecules, which are part of the cellular membrane, act as anchoring points for the extracellular matrix and for the microtubules in the cytoskeleton.

The impact of this was huge: Dr Ingber's research group for the Children's Vascular Biology Program at Harvard University successfully proved that a mechanical force applied to a tissue is sensed first by the integrins at the anchor points and then propagated deep into each cell by the cytoskeleton. Once inside, this force can vibrate or change the shape of the protein molecule by activating a biochemical reaction or even stimulate a chromosome inside the nucleus, thus activating a gene. 'Ingber says that cells also have 'tone,' just like muscles, because of the constant pull of the cytoskeletal filaments. Much as a stretched violin string produces different sounds when force is applied at different points along its length, the cell processes chemical signals differently depending on how much it is distorted' (Fliesler, n.d.).

Let us return to the collagen fiber, the 'clearly hollow' (Guimberteau, 2005) and liquid-filled (CSF?) armature of the matrix which is directly linked to the microtubules of the cytoskeleton by way of the integrins. What could they be exchanging? Beyond the possibility that the CSF is penetrating the cells through the microtubules, it is a relief to read that science has found that the simple mechanical action of touching a living tissue can have such a profound effect that it can even influence the DNA.

Ingber concluded his article 'Mechanochemical basis of cell and tissue regulation' with a phrase which would have pleased Andrew T. Still: 'The riddle of how cells form specialized tissues and organs is more a problem in structural design, systems engineering, and architecture, than a question of chemistry. Because the hierarchical molecular structures that comprise living cells, tissues, and organs are stabilized based on tensegrity principles, cells are perfectly poised to sense physical signals, to respond mechanically, and to orchestrate a spatially coordinated biochemical response at the molecular level. For this reason, **structure dictates function in living cells' (Ingber, 2004).**

# APPENDIX V

## What the therapist can observe during and after a still point

### James Jealous DO:

'[...] all of a sudden, you will feel a long inhalation and the patient will take in a deep breath involuntarily which is completely synchronized with a similar deep breath in primary respiration. All of a sudden, the boundaries of the inhalation phase dissolve and the patient is breathing thoracic and primary respiration together and synchronized, and you have even more augmentation. And after that, things get very very quiet, usually there is a still point. It comes to a point of balance and rests for a while. In a neutral; it is not breathing in, it is not breathing out. It is just there, balanced upon the stillness from which it emerged at conception. If you are successful with that EV4, it is going to take a number of days for that treatment to really sink in' (Jealous, 2000, Expansion of the fourth ventricle [EV4] No 1, track 17).

### Pierre Tricot DO:

'Mechanical reharmonization: the area which was retracted alters the deep body tissue mechanics, meaning that modifications and mechanical compensations must set in. As the retention which made them necessary disappears or decreases, the body itself must also modify its adaptive or compensatory mechanisms. Since, however, it has been able to create them in order to adapt to an anomaly, it is also able to stop creating them when they are no longer needed.

'From a biological point of view, the area which was hyperfunctioning recovers normal activity enabling it to assume more correctly its physiology. The body is thus relieved and finds a more normal functioning. The release of retention also releases various substances which were trapped in the region due to the stagnation of microcirculation. The release of these substances into circulation may explain the patient's perception of taste or odor, and the fatigue experienced in the days following a session.

'Return to consciousness: Restoration of communication in the region leads to its reintegration in the body's consciousness pattern. The patient often verbalizes this by expressing that he now feels as if that part of the body is alive, whereas before, he paid it little attention or indeed ignored it. The patient may also recover memories corresponding to the event which had caused the retention, despite having said at the first visit that he did not recall any event, traumatic or otherwise, which may have created it' (Tricot, 2005, p. 118).

Encoding of tactile forces in the primary somatosensory cortex

Pascal Fortier-Poisson, University of Montreal, April 2012

The following passage was taken from Pascal Fortier-Poisson's doctoral thesis in neurological sciences:

> Modulation of S1 is influenced by certain cortical mechanisms such as attention (Chapman, 1994). Thus, the overall activity of S1 is increased if the monkey must discriminate surfaces slid under his finger rather than endure them while performing a visual or auditory task (Hsiao et al., 1993; Burton and Sinclair, 2000; Chapman and Meftah, 2005). A task in which the animal must be attentive to a stimulus applied to the skin gives a strong response in S1. (Fortier-Poisson, 2012, p. 20)

S1 is the primary somatosensory cortex. It receives very dense afferents from the thalamus and its neurons respond intensely to somatosensory stimuli (but very little to noxious stimuli).[1]

Lesions in S1 impair somatic sensation and electrical stimulation of this cortical area evokes somatic sensory experiences (Bear, Connors and Paradiso, 2007, p.401).

Indeed, electrical stimulation of the surface of the S1 area may be the origin of somatic sensations susceptible to be localized precisely to different parts of the body, depending on the exact site of the stimulation.

We find ourselves faced with some questions:

–We know that stimulation of cutaneous mechanoreceptors activates the S1 area. We know that the stimulation of S1 can produce sensations at a specific site according to the S1 zone stimulated and that the activity of the primary sensory cortex will be increased if it is allowed to pay attention to the applied skin stimulus. In addition to the pause that we recommend, should we ask the patient to focus on what he feels and should we eliminate all forms of stimulation (phone, talking with the patient, odors such as essential oils or incense, cold and too bright lighting)?

–Then, when the skin is no longer being touched and the person continues to feel something in his body, for example tingling, heat, or a feeling that 'energy' is flowing, we know, thanks to Dr Craig, that this is an activation of the insular cortex. Could there be a reverberating circuit phenomenon in the area of the insular cortex which prolongs the feeling? Is it not better to wait until the sensation has attenuated before touching the patient again?

We do not know at this time, but we know that if we touch the patient again, his attention will be drawn to these new stimuli and that there a risk of inhibiting the preceding stimuli. When in doubt, would it not be better to abstain and simply create a pause?

### Note

[1.] 'Complete removal of the somatic sensory areas of the cerebral cortex does not destroy an animal's ability to perceive pain. Therefore, it is likely that pain impulses entering the brain stem reticular formation, the thalamus and other lower brain centers cause conscious perception of pain. This does not mean that the cerebral cortex has nothing to do with normal pain appreciation; electrical stimulation of cortical somatosensory areas does cause a human being to perceive mild pain from about 3 percent of the points stimulated. However, it is believed that the cortex plays an especially important role in interpreting pain quality, even though pain perception might be principally the function of lower centers (Hall and Guyton, 2011)'. As we saw in the chapter on homeostasis, Craig situates the perception of information center coming from primary afferent A∂ and C-fibers, including nociceptors, in the anterior insular cortex (Craig, 2015).

# AFTERWORD

'Osteopathic ideas come slowly. We do right to scrutinize carefully the new ideas our people advance that we may avoid accepting anything footless or fantastic. On the other hand, our latitude for the entertainment of a new theory or interpretation is great, because we are exploring a field new even to us - a field given scant consideration by the so-called standard therapeutic investigators. We need not fear giving full consideration to new ideas advanced by our people. (MacDonald, 1932, cited in Sutherland, 1939, reprinted 2015, p.13).

John A. MacDonald DO

Past-President, American Osteopathic Association

The innovative nature of somatosensory integration time can be confusing: there is nothing new, however; it had simply to be brought to light.

Having been recognized and named, it is now time to give it the place it deserves.

# REFERENCES

Barral, J.P., 2004. *Manipulations viscérales 1*. 2nd ed. Paris: Elsevier.

Barrett, K., Barman, S.M., Boitano, S., Brooks, H.L., 2010. *Ganong's Review of Medical Physiology*. 23rd ed. New York: McGraw-Hill Medical.

Bear, M.F., Connors, B.W. and Paradiso, M.A., 2007. *Neuroscience, Exploring the Brain*. Baltimore: Lippincott Williams & Wilkins.

Becker, R.E., 2001. *The Stillness of Life*. Edited by Rachel E. Brooks. Portland, OR: Stillness Press.

Becker, R.E., 2006. *Life in Motion*. Edited by Rachel E. Brooks. Portland, OR: Rachel E. Brooks.

Branly, R. [n.d.] *Reasoned Osteopathy*. Available at: http://www.niromathe.com/down_public/niromathe_book_en.pdf [Accessed June 22, 2015]

Burton, H. and Sinclair R.J., 2000. Tactile-spatial and cross-modal attention effects in the primary somatosensory cortical areas 3b and 1-2 of rhesus monkeys 2. *Somatosens Mot Res* 17: 213–228.

Campbell, S.S. and Murphy, P.J., 1998. *Extraocular Circadian Phototransduction in Humans*. *Science*, January 16; 279 (5349):396–399.

Chapman, C.E., 1994. Active versus passive touch: factors influencing the transmission of somatosensory signals to primary somatosensory cortex 4. *Can J Physiol Pharmacol* 72: 558–570.

Chapman, C.E. and Meftah, E.M., 2005. Independent controls of attentional influences in primary and secondary somatosensory cortex. *J Neurophysiol* 94: 4094–4107.

Chauffour, P. and Prat E., 2002. *Mechanical Links*. Berkeley: North Atlantic Books.

Craig, A.D., 2002. How do you feel? Interoception: the sense of the physiological condition of the body. *Nature Reviews Neuroscience*; 3: 655–666. Available at: www.nature.com/nrn/journal/v3/n8/full/nrn894.html [Accessed June 23, 2015]

Craig, A.D., 2003. Pain mechanisms: labeled lines versus convergence in central processing. *Annual Reviews Neuroscience*; 26:1–30. Available at:

http://www.annualreviews.org/doi/pdf/10.1146/annurev.neuro.
26.041002.131022 [Accessed June 23, 2015]

Craig, A.D., 2009. How do you feel? The neuroanatomical basis for human awareness of feelings from the body: right/left asymmetry. [video] Lecture by Bud Craig at the Linköping Universitet. Available at: https://vimeo.com/8170544 [Accessed June 23, 2015]

Craig, A.D., 2015. *How do you feel? An Interoceptive Moment with your Neurobiological Self*. Princeton, NJ: Princeton University Press.

Croibier, A., 2005. *Diagnostic ostéopathique général*. Paris: Elsevier.

Cross, S. J. and Albury, W.R., 1987. Walter B. Cannon, L.J. Henderson, and the organic analogy. *Osiris*; 3(2):165–172. Available at: http://www.jstor.org/discover/10.2307/301758?uid=3739464&uid=2&uid=3737720&uid=4&sid=21106685579833 [Accessed June 23, 2015]

Duval, J.A., 2008. *Techniques ostéopathiques d'équilibre et d'échanges réciproques*. Vannes: Sully.

Early American Manual Therapy. http://www.mcmillinmedia.com/eamt/files/contents.htm [Accessed June 23, 2015]

Fernandez, D. and Lecine, A.,1988. *Cinésiologie du rein*, Aix-en-Provence: CREDO.

Fliesler, N. [n.d.] The mechanical cell. Dream magazine, published by Boston Children's Hospital.

Fortier-Poisson, P., 2012. Encodage des forces tactiles dans le cortex somatosensoriel primaire. Université de Montréal, Faculté des études supérieures, PhD. © Pascal Fortier-Poisson. Available at: https://papyrus.bib.umontreal.ca/xmlui/bitstream/handle/1866/8619/Fortier-Poisson_Pascal_2012_these.pdf?sequence=2 [Accessed June 23, 2015]

Furness, J.B., 2007. The enteric nervous system, *Scholarpedia*; 2(10):4064. Available at: http://www.scholarpedia.org/article/Enteric_nervous_system [Accessed June 23, 2015]

Gastaldi, G. and Ruiz, J., 2009. Dysfonction métabolique et stress chronique: un nouveau regard sur la pandémie de 'diabésité'? *Revue Médicale Suisse*; 206:1273–1277. Available at: http://www.revmed.ch/

rms/2009/RMS-206/Dysfonction-metabolique et-stress-chronique-un-nouveau-regard-sur-la-pandemie-de-diabesite [Accessed June 23, 2015]

Gershon, M.D., 1998. *The Second Brain*. New York: HarperCollins.

Godefroid, J., 2008. *Psychologie: science humaine et cognitive*. Brussels: de Boeck.

Gravett, H.H., 1948. Echoes from Dr. Still's lectures to the class of ninety six. *Academy of Applied Osteopathy Yearbook*; 1948:48–51.

Gregory, A.E., 1922. *Spondylotherapy Simplified*. Early American Manual Therapy. Available at: http://www.mcmillinmedia.com/eamt/files/gregory/gregcont.htm [Accessed June 23, 2015]

Grosjean, D., 1984. *Traité pratique de microkinésithérapie, tome 1*. 1re ed. Pont-à-Mousson: CFM

Grosjean, D., 2014. Exchange of emails in June 2014.

Guimberteau, J-C., 2005. *Strolling under the skin*. DVD Vanves: ADF Vidéo production.

Hall, J. E. and Guyton, A.C., 2011. *Guyton and Hall Textbook of Medical Physiology*. 12th ed. Philadelphia: Saunders, Elsevier.

Hsiao, S.S., O'Shaughnessy, D.M. and Johnson, K.O., 1993. Effects of selective attention on spatial form processing in monkey primary and secondary somatosensory cortex. *J.Neurophysiol*. 70: 444–447.

Ingber, D., 2004. *Mechanochemical Basis of Cell and Tissue Regulation*. Washington: *The Bridge: Linking Engineering and Society*, 34; (3): 4–10.

Jacobs, D., 2009. *Dermoneuromodulation treatment manual*. [self-published]

Jacobs, D., 2012. *Dermoneuromodulation: What?! .. ANOTHER 'technique'??* Available at: http://forwardthinkingpt.com/2012/03/12/dermoneuromodulation-what-another-technique/ [Accessed June 23, 2015]

Jealous, J., 2000. The biodynamics of osteopathy. [CDs] Apollo Beach, FL: Marnee Jealous Long.

Jones, L.H., 1995. *Strain-CounterStrain*. Boise, ID: Boise Jones Strain-CounterStrain Inc.

Kamina, P., 2008. *Anatomie clinique, tome 5*. Paris: Maloine.

Kohn, M.I., Tanna, N.K., Herman, G.T., et al., 1991. Analysis of the brain and cerebrospinal fluid volumes with MR imaging: impact of PET data correction for atrophy. *Radiology*, Jan; 178(1):115–22.

Korr, I.M., 1947. The neural basis of the osteopathic lesion. *The Journal of the American Osteopathic Association*; 47(4).

Laget, P. [n.d.] Somesthésie. *Encyclopédie universalis* [online]. Subchapter on 'Sensory modalities'. Available at: www.universalis.fr/encyclopedie/somesthesie [Accessed June 24, 2015]

Lane, M.A, 1925, *Doctor A.T. Still: Founder of Osteopathy*. Available at: https://archive.org/stream/dratstillfounder00lane#page/24/mode/2up [Accessed June 24, 2015]

Lazorthes, G., 1973. *Le système nerveux central: description, systématisation, exploration*. Paris: Masson et Cie.

Lazorthes, G., 1986. *L'ouvrage des sens*. Paris: Flammarion.

LeDoux, J., 2002. *Synaptic Self: How our Brains Become Who We Are*. [e-book] Toronto: Vicking.

Lehouelleur, J., 2015. Introduction à la physiologie – notion d'homéostasie. Available at: www.neur-one.fr [Accessed June 24, 2015]

Magoun, H.I., 1976. *Osteopathy in the Cranial Field*. 3rd ed. Produced under the auspices of The Cranial Academy Inc. Harold Ives Magoun, Sr.

Manent, J.B. [n.d.] Les bases neuronales de la mémoire: ou comment les neurones stockent-ils nos souvenirs? Marseille: Institut de Neurobiologie de la Méditerranée, INMED/INSERM U29.

Marieb, E.N., 1993. *Anatomie et physiologie humaine*. Montreal: Éditions du renouveau pédagogique.

McEwen, B.S., 2002. *The End of Stress As We Know It*. Washington: Joseph Henri Press.

McEwen, B.S., 2007. Physiology and neurobiology of stress and adaptation: central role of the brain. *Physiological Review*; 87(3):873–904. Available at: http://physrev.physiology.org/content/87/3/873.full#BIBL [Accessed June 24, 2015]

McEwen, B.S. and Wingfield, J.C., 2003. The concept of allostasis in biology and biomedicine. *Hormones and Behavior*; 43:2–15. Available through Science Direct website: www.sciencedirect.com [Accessed June 24, 2015]

Odent, M., 2002. *The Farmer and the Obstetrician*. London: Free Association Books Limited.

Palmer, B. J., 1936. *The Known Man*. Davenport: The Palmer School of Chiropractic.

Paulus, S., 2009. Exploring the philosophy of osteopathy: find it, fix it, leave it alone. Was available at: www.interlinea.org in 2009.

Racano, P., 2014. Comments added during the correction of the 2014 version.

Robbins, T., 1986. *Unlimited Powers*. New York: Simon & Schuster Paperbacks, New York.

Robitaille, R., 2009. Comments added during the correction of the 2009 version.

Rose, D., 2004. *Les neurobranchés: les systèmes sensoriels*. Available at: http://neurobranches.chez-alice.fr [Accessed June 24, 2015]

Saine, F., 1996. *Les différences et les similitudes entre la chiropratique et l'ostéopathie*. Montreal: Collège d'Études Ostéopathiques.

Sauvanet, P., 2000. *Le rythme et la raison*. Paris: Kimé.

Sergueef, N., Nelson, K.E. and Glonek, T., 2001. Les modifications de l'onde de Traube–Hering après traitement crânien (Changes in the Traube Hering wave following cranial manipulation). *The American Academy of Osteopathy Journal*; 11(1).

Snow, A., 1912. Mechanical vibration. Available on the Early American Manual Therapy website at: http://www.mcmillinmedia.com/eamt/files/snow/mvcont.htm [Accessed June 24, 2015]

Stark, J.E., 2012. Quoting A.T. Still with rigor: an historical and academic review. *The Journal of the American Osteopathic Association*; 112(6).

Sutherland, A.S., 1962. *With Thinking Fingers: The Story of William Garner Sutherland*. The Cranial Academy.

Sutherland, W.G., 1939. *The Cranial Bowl*. Reprinted 2015. The Osteopathic Cranial Academy. Indianopolis, USA.

Sutherland, W.G., 1998. *Contributions of Thoughts: The Collected Writings of William Garner Sutherland*. 2nd ed. Edited by Adah Strand Sutherland and Anne L. Wales. Sutherland Cranial Teaching Foundation Inc.

Tortora, G.J. and Derrickson, B., 2009. *Principles of Anatomy and Physiology*. 12th ed. USA: John Wiley and Sons Inc.

Tortora, G.J. and Grabowski, S.R., 2001. *Principes d'anatomie et de physiologie*. Ville Saint-Laurent: ERPI.

Tremblay, L., 2007. *The Little Bowen Book*. Montreal: Éditions Louise Tremblay

Tricot, P. [n.d.] Article on A.T. Still's conference at the American School of Osteopathy in 1896. This article, translated by Pierre Tricot, can be found on the website: www.approche-tissulaire.fr [Accessed June 20, 2015]

Tricot, P., 2005. *Approche tissulaire de l'ostéopathie*, Vannes: Sully.

Tricot, P., 2009. From a letter to Louise Tremblay, July 20, 2009.

Upledger, J.E. and Vredevoogd, J.D., 2014 [1983]. *Craniosacral Therapy*. Seattle: Eastland Press.

Vibert, J.F., 2007. *Circuits et réseaux de neurones, bruit, traitement de l'information*, [pdf] Paris: Faculté de Médecine Pierre et Marie Curie, Paris.

Waugh, A. and Grant, A., 2010. *Ross and Wilson: Anatomy and Physiology in Health and Illness*. 11th ed. Churchill Livingstone.

# FURTHER READING

Ferreira, B., 2009. *Jones strain-counterstrain : une technique manuelle au service de la kinésithérapie.* MKDE. Available at: http://www.kine-formations.com/Jones-strain-counterstrain-mode-d-action_a413.html [Accessed June 23, 2015]

Lever, R., 2013. *At the Still Point of the Turning World - the art and philosophy of osteopathy.* Edinburgh: Handspring Publishing.

Misery, L., 2000. *La peau neuronale, les nerfs à fleur de peau.* Paris: Éditions Ellipses.

Paoletti, S., 2005. *Les fascias: rôle des tissus dans la mécanique humaine.* Vannes: Éditions Sully.

Paris, C. and Bastarache, Y., 1995. *Philosopher: pensée critique et argumentation.* Quebec: Éditions C.G. Inc.

Reinberg, A., 2003. *Chronobiologie médicale: chrono-thérapeutique.* Paris: Flammarion.

Sherrington, C.S., 1948. *The Integrative Action of the Nervous System.* Cambridge: Cambridge University Press.

Still, A.T., 1910. *Osteopathy, Research and Practice.* Kirksville, MO: The author.

Widmaier, E.P., Raff, H. and Strang, K.T., 2010. *Vander's Human Physiology: The Mechanisms of Body Function.* 12th ed. McGraw-Hill Higher Education.

# INDEX

**Note:** Page number followed by f indicates figure only.

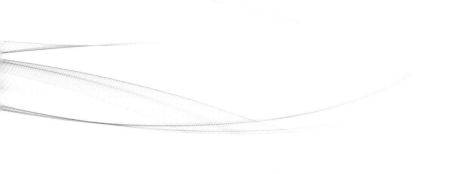

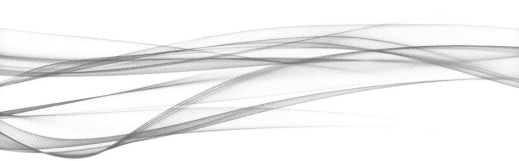

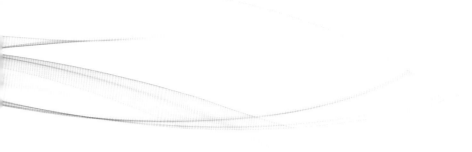